O₂XYGEN THERAPIES

A NEW WAY OF AF...

BY ED McCABE

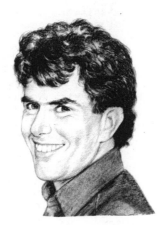

ENERGY PUBLICATIONS

99-RD1 MORRISVILLE, NY 13408 U.S.A.

TITLE: O$_2$XYGEN THERAPIES

KEYWORDS: OXYGEN, OXYGENATION, HYDROGEN PEROXIDE, PEROXIDE, OZONE, PHOTOZONE, AEROX, STABILIZED OXYGEN, AEROBIC 07, GERMANIUM, CO-Q10, SUPEROXIDE DISMUTASE,   ACIDOPHILUS,   LIPIDS,   HYDROXY PEROXIDES, PEROXISOMES,   CATALASE,   AIDS,   CANCER,   ARTHRITIS,   CANDIDIASIS, DIABETES, LUKEMIA, MULTIPLE SCLEROSIS, MUTATING, VIRUSES, MICROBES, BACTERIA,   PATHOGENS,   HEALTH,   POOLS,   SPAS,   TOXIC   WASTE, MUNICIPAL DRINKING WATER, AGRICULTURE.

Illustrated by: Betsy Bullard

Editorial, and other assistance, generously provided by:
Marjorie Bousquet
Dot Bullard
Dr. Larry Preble
Gerry Price
Richard Taub
Michael Schwartz
Marlene Avery Westcott
Hi, Neighbor Staff
Desmark
Kyocera
On-Line Store

Other assistance by:
Loosie & Flow

Printed in U.S.A.

Library of Congress Catalog Card Number: 88-81291

ISBN: 0-9620527-0-1 $15

THIS BOOK EXISTS IN THE NAME OF SUGMAD

MY FRIEND, AND MORE.

WE CAN DO ANYTHING UNLESS WE BELIEVE WE CAN'T

CONSCIOUSNESS IS EVERYTHING

TABLE OF CONTENTS

HYDROGEN PEROXIDE

OZONE O_3

PILLS, PRODUCTS, PLACES
PROPOSALS, & PATHS

ABOUT THE AUTHOR'S EXPERIENCES

My nature is synthesis, analysis, and communication. I earned my degree in Educational Media from the University of Massachusetts and set out to increase my knowledge by personal investigation.

I always have had to know, "WHY?". My knowledge of healing systems kept growing during my pursuit of truth. I studied most of our world's spiritual teachings. As I went around searching for the Divinity within me, I also discovered many types of healing.

During the past 18 years, I have studied many healing ways, and read piles of books on alternative and mainstream healing practices. I've corresponded, stayed with, interviewed, and learned from mainstream orthodox and also relatively unknown spiritual teachers and health care professionals. I tried many of the methods myself and gained direct experience. I discarded methods of a lesser efficiency, while incorporating those that worked for me into my base of knowledge. Perhaps some of what I learned can work for you.

Most importantly, in the healing area, I discovered that there is a triad of concerns that need to be balanced before real long term healing can be effected:

```
                           *
                        MENTAL

                  *           *

              *                   *
                    SPIRITUAL
              *                   *

    PHYSICAL    *     *     *   EMOTIONAL
```

Above and beyond these areas, as if you are looking down on the top of a pyramid, The SPIRITUAL is the invisible thread that ties them all together yet remains apart from their dualistic natures. For us to be in harmony, all four need to be faced, examined, and balanced.

You won't be healthy long if you abuse your body in the areas of food, drugs, rest, breath, or exercise, or if you give in to excessive anger, lust, greed, attachment, or vanity. You also won't be healthy long if you dwell upon thinking badly about yourself or others, or deliberately, somehow, reduce or abberate your incoming and outgoing flow of the LIFE FORCE.

If you do these things, whether by conscious choice or not, disease and suffering follow. If not right away, then eventually, as it is Nature's way of getting you to wake up and see how you are BEING, as part of the WHOLE.

WHY I WROTE THIS BOOK

About three years ago, in the magazine "The Journal of Borderland Research" I read about German doctors eliminating the AIDS virus in patients by ozonation of their blood. The Europeans have used ozone for over 30 years. I then began reading about Father Willhelm and his student, Walter Grotz's combined efforts promoting Hydrogen Peroxide as a detoxifier and healer. I got their tapes and tried it on myself. I spoke with people (some over 70) who have used it for 5 years. This led me to the work of Tom Valentine, Aerox, and his family of oxygenation products. Then I heard of Terrence McGrath, who started a public ozone treatment company in the U.S. called, Medizone. Medizone had secured a patent, FDA "I.N.D." (Investigative New Drug) Status, and built a substantial corporate base. Next came all the oxygenation enhancers and supplements and their proponents. During this time I noticed the large number of followers that all the above-mentioned oxygenation methods started attracting, and larger numbers of case histories of thankful people started appearing. I noticed that there was no one book that spelled out all the methods under one cover, compared them, presented scientific documentation on them, and told where they came from. Hopefully this work fills that gap.

"O$_2$XYGEN THERAPIES" IS AIMED AT THREE LEVELS

Level 1. Everyday mainstream busy people who don't follow science much, summed up by the question once posed to me: "People in Europe have AIDS?" These readers are advised to skip-read the technical sections written for level 3. Use what you can, and wait for the video.

Level 2. The level of seasoned, informed, alternative health care "hobbyists" and seekers who are knowledgeable but under-informed in this area or need a reference to make a point. This would be all the "healthfood store customers" and "exercise" types.

Level 3. This level is for the Medical professional. Someone wanting to educate someone else who is a health professional, or someone doing an educational research paper. I have included the full technical medical descriptions of the oxygenation processes for them. I have also supplied numerous references to encourage further study and investigation. Note: to make this book easily readable and even enjoyable by people at level 1, at times I had to depart from an airtight "guarded" medical presentation. If you read this and find yourself saying "That statement wasn't scientific.", it wasn't written for your level, and please contact the European doctors, or Dr. Farr, Dr. Sunnen, or Dr. Freibott, for example (contacts at end of book), who will speak a more professional language to you. Please do not discount the proven oxidation processes, due to any of my literary shortcomings.

WHY THIS BOOK WAS WRITTEN ON MANY LEVELS

Any of my friends whom I told I was, "writing a book about people who drink hydrogen peroxide" have given me the same strange look and said, "people drink it"...? I then explain how it is found in mothers milk, our immune systems, our intestines, rainwater, and all the healing springs around the world. Still looking at me like I'm crazy, they don't seem to relax until I quickly add that "Oh, not the kind in the drug store, I mean FOOD GRADE hydrogen peroxide." When I say "ozone", I see what a great job of disinformation and bad science the media has done, since "everyone knows it's smog". They even have scientists who know it isn't, calling pollution "ozone" on the news.

So, my work is to not only to present you with the wonders that are possible with oxygenation but to prove to you that it is a scientifically credible subject as well. To this end, I have filled this work with scientific documentation. Sprinkled throughout the quotes and references are a lot of big words with which you may feel only a "rocket scientist" would be comfortable Since well-meaning medical professionals who haven't done any research on our subject may be skeptical, and require documentation, I have included everything scientific right along with the stories. You may think some of this subject is not light reading, but you should have seen it before I translated a lot of it into an "everyday" level!

The words that you don't get, either look up or skip. Either way, there's plenty of **worthwhile** *material in-between.*

This book is worth studying. The information in it may someday save your life or the life of someone you love (or at least make them more comfortable). Most everyone I know seems to get sick more often these days. It's just as true that most everyone I know who has tried oxygenating their cells through one of the methods in this book has improved, substantially or slightly, if he stayed with it. Keep an open mind, an adventurous spirit, and you may be pleasantly surprised!

The information in here may also show your community how to; clean up a toxic waste dump, restore a wildlife habitat, or purify your municipal drinking water supply. Or perhaps you can tell your neighbor how to get that chlorine smell out of his pool, hot tub, or spa, saving money, and at the same time have even purer water. How can all this be related? OXYGEN!

How can I get the message of restoring missing oxygen to scientists and normal everyday people alike? We all; breathe, drink water, and have concerns about toxic waste. I'm not sure, but this book attempts to show how this has been accomplished, and our lives may depend upon it someday.

Something for everyone, we all can work together.

MY OXYGENATION EXPERIENCES

I started by ingesting a few drops of diluted 35% solution of food-grade hydrogen peroxide in juice two or three times a day. Ignoring the "bleachy taste" and uneasy feeling, I knew it was breaking down into water and oxygen in my system. I did this for four months. The first thing that happened was that my intestines emptied accumulated waste-matter heavily for three days. A few weeks went by as I slowly increased the dosage, and then I came down with a fever for two weeks. A week went by and then I started coughing and expectorating. This lasted for about two months.

I investigated these reactions by speaking with people who had more oxygenation experiences than I. I kept hearing about, and reading of, the same viewpoint, and I personally found this viewpoint to be the most logical: My body finally had enough oxygen in it to clean itself out. This viewpoint was also backed up with, and based upon, the cleansing reactions I have had in the past, during fasting and the use of other cleansing products.

I am not a scientist, and I had no scientific way to measure anything that happened to me, but since it is my body, I have an intuitive and logical opinion as to the sequence of events I experienced. I now assume this is what happened to me: First, my intestines started dumping out toxins, much like a colonic or enema. This could have included many forms of freshly expired anaerobic bacteria. Then the individual body cells began to be oxygenated, dumping out their own accumulated toxins. My metabolic rate increased to the point of fever, to burn up these toxins for elimination.

Then the extra oxygen released into my bloodstream started to bubble out of the blood in the air/blood exchange area of my lung bronchial sacs. This happened underneath the coatings of accumulated toxins left over from my many bouts of childhood bronchitis. The layers loosened, and as they broke up, I expelled them. Other people have had other cleansing reactions such as rashes, or none at all, depending on how clean their cells were when they started. I have since found out that I could have avoided some of the unpleasant reactions by first cleansing my colon. I believe the reactions were all beneficial, because I have not been sick since. I used to get the flu and colds constantly.

Since then, I've been using Aerox, and Aerobic 07. Both are saline solutions of sodium chlorite, which carry electrolytes of oxygen into the blood via the stomach. I now also take SOD/antioxidant complexes. I alternate Aerox with rubbed-into-my-skin aloe & hydrogen peroxide gel and Body Toddy. I also cleaned out my colon, and use Homozone, a Magnesium based powdered ozone carrier, as well as Biotene hydrogen peroxide producing toothpaste. All these products are detailed in different sections of the book.

Here are my "side effects" or results, since the cleansing, they're given to you with my intuitive/subjective conclusions:

I need less sleep each night. Sleep is when our bodies eliminate the waste products from the day's activities, so I must not need as much cleaning.

So far, I have not had a cold or flu in over 2 years, where I used to be sick approximately 4 times a year. Apparently anaerobic cold & flu viruses can't stand my new cellular oxygen level, and I have fewer internal "swamps" for them to grow in. I hope this trend continues, but if I do get sick, then it doesn't automatically discount the effectiveness of oxygenation. Perhaps It means that some other area of my life is out of balance.

I haven't had to go to a chiropractor in two years, other than once, because of a direct physical injury. Before, my old spine, neck, and pelvic conditions were increasingly "going out" and requiring constant treatment. These increasingly frequent painful events were probably due to the aging process of arthritic spurs growing on my joints. I saw them on x-rays. I don't know exactly why this is, but I assume metabolic waste toxins and microbes in my joints are being oxidized and eliminated, and my connective tissues are regaining flexibility. Any microbes that were living in my cells and creating waste product build up, are also being oxidized and eliminated. I also have fewer and lesser allergic reactions now, my hay fever has stopped, and my normal ear wax has increased, after being dried up for years.

CAUTIONARY STATEMENT AND DISCLAIMER

THE AUTHOR IS A REPORTER, NOT A DOCTOR. WHAT YOU DO WITH THIS INFORMATION IS UP TO YOU AND NOT HIS RESPONSIBILITY. The following true statement is mandated by current laws, Postal and FDA directives.

WARNING: THIS BOOK IS SOLD FOR EDUCATIONAL AND RESEARCH PURPOSES ONLY. ANY OF THE INFORMATION IMPARTED HEREIN IS NOT MEDICAL ADVICE, DIAGNOSIS OR PRESCRIPTION. YOU ARE WARNED TO SEEK HEALING SOLUTIONS FROM QUALIFIED HEALTH CARE PROFESSIONALS. SELF TREATMENT CAN BE HAZARDOUS IF SOMEONE HAS A SERIOUS AILMENT.

THE AUTHOR/PUBLISHER/PRINTER IS NOT RESPONSIBLE FOR DAMAGES OR OTHER LIABILITIES. HE CANNOT GUARANTEE THE ACCURACY, SAFETY OR EFFECTIVENESS OF THE DATA GATHERED AND PRESENTED WITHIN THIS WORK.

NOTHING HEREIN IS INTENDED TO OFFEND ANY PERSON OR GROUP, OR TO IMPLY OR INFER THE BREAKING OF ANY LAWS OR AGENCY DIRECTIVES. THIS BOOK IS NOT PRACTICING MEDICINE WITHOUT A LICENSE, ILLEGAL ADVERTISING, LABELING, MAIL FRAUD, LIBEL OR IN ANY WAY INTENDED TO BE DISRUPTIVE TO OUR PRESENT DAY HEALTHCARE DELIVERY SYSTEM. FOR CRITICAL INJURIES AND SOME ACUTE DISEASES, ORTHODOX THERAPY IS MORE EFFECTIVE. THIS BOOK IS ONLY A HISTORICAL CHRONICLE OF THE PAST AND PRESENT SOCIAL AND SCIENTIFIC USE OF, AND RESEARCH WITH, OXYGENATION PROCESSES AND PRODUCTS. THE AUTHOR OR EDITOR OR PUBLISHER OR PRINTER OR DISTRIBUTORS OR RETAIL OUTLETS TAKE NO LEGAL RESPONSIBILITY WHATSOEVER FOR THE CONTENTS WITHIN.

ALTHOUGH QUALIFIED HISTORICAL STUDIES HAVE, TO THIS POINT, SHOWN NONTOXICITY AT PROPER DOSAGE LEVELS, THE POTENT OXIDIZERS AS DISCUSSED IN THIS WORK, IF APPLIED INCORRECTLY, OR IN TOO STRONG A CONCENTRATION, CAN OXIDIZE (BURN) HEALTHY BODY CELLS AND TISSUE.

EXAMPLES OF POSSIBLE HARM:

UNLIKE THE REGULAR DRUGSTORE 3% STRENGTH, IF YOU SPILL UNDILUTED 35% SOLUTION FOOD-GRADE HYDROGEN PEROXIDE ON YOUR SKIN, IT WILL IMMEDIATELY TURN WHITE, BURN, AND STING FOR DAYS. DRINKING IT WOULD DO SERIOUS HARM. NEVER USE UNDILUTED HYDROGEN PEROXIDE INTERNALLY OR EXTERNALLY. OBSERVE ALL PRECAUTIONS. KEEP OUT OF THE REACH OF CHILDREN. UNDILUTED 35% LOOKS JUST LIKE WATER AND A CHILD COULD DRINK IT BY MISTAKE. ALWAYS STORE IT IN BOLDLY MARKED TAMPER-PROOF CONTAINERS THAT DON'T LOOK LIKE NORMAL DRINKS.

IF YOU BREATHE CONCENTRATED OZONE, ESPECIALLY IF IT'S IN A CONTAMINATED FORM (SEE TEXT), INTO YOUR LUNGS, OR GET IT ON SENSITIVE MEMBRANES, IT CAN DAMAGE YOU. EVEN GETTING TOO CLOSE TO A ROOM IONIZER COULD IRRITATE YOUR THROAT.

PLEASE BE CAREFUL

HYDROGEN PEROXIDE

PIONEERING PEROXIDE PROMOTERS

We're going to start the book with excerpts from talks given by four different hydrogen peroxide proponents. They will show how nature has provided many ways of supplying us oxygen carrying hydrogen peroxide for our use. We'll also see the many ways experimental science is proving that cellular oxygen levels are important to health. Any comments I make in this section will be preceded by "Note:" Anything else will be the particular speaker's experiences and opinions.

WILLHELM AND GROTZ INTRODUCED

Reverend Father Richard Willhelm, from Naples, FL, many years ago, understood the possibilities of hydrogen peroxide. Here was a man who had dedicated his life to a calling, taught physics, and understood the basics. These truths were so evident to him that he began wanting to discuss them and throughout his years talked to many different individuals. Some laughed at him, some scoffed him, some denigrated his mental ability and wondered about premature senility, yet he kept on.

Then one time he met a person who was to become a faithful disciple; Walter Grotz, a retired postmaster. Of all individuals to take up a banner; a retired postmaster! Wally Grotz listened to Father Willhelm and said he would try using hydrogen peroxide on his arthritis. The hydrogen peroxide worked and Wally Grotz said "Thank you Father Willhelm, I had great response from that and I will go on with my life". Wally Grotz said it was great and he wanted to tell others about it. He did, he began to tell others.

On January 18, 1987, The National Health Federation held their 32nd Annual Convention, in Pasadena, California. The NHF awarded it's 1987 Pioneer Award to Father Richard Willhelm and Walter O. Grotz for having discovered and shared the healing properties of hydrogen peroxide. The NHF "is proud to honor men who, like the pioneers of old, have gone forward into uncharted waters and stood the winds of ridicule and have seen those who ridiculed them change and become proponents. Walter O. Grotz and Father Richard Willhelm are indeed true pioneers".

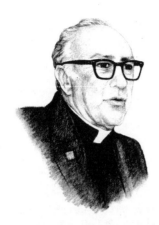

FATHER RICHARD WILLHELM, B.S.

THE MAN WHO PUBLICLY STARTED IT ALL

The world owes a debt to medical men like Dr. Murray and Dr. Rosenow for their pioneering research, but it would have collected dust in the medical libraries if not for the work of Father Richard Willhelm, and his prize student Walter Grotz. Following them, and equally deserving of our thanks, are Dr. Farr and Dr. Donsbach.

Note: From here to the end of this section, I will be quoting from public addresses given by these four men.

Father Willhelm: I'm glad that Walter Grotz is here. I call him my disciple. I've been doing work with ozone and hydrogen peroxide ever since I've been ordained and we're awfully glad people are listening to us and finding out that this is God's own way to keep us germ free and bacteria free. Right after I was ordained 43 years ago, I became interested in ozone.

DRS. MURRAY & McCLELLEN

I generated ozone for Dr. Maynard Murray, and we bubbled ozone through blood back in 1944-45. The real reason I got interested in the peroxide is that there was a Dr. Harold McClellen in Dayton, who was trying to find a bacteriological cause of mental illness. I sat up nights talking with him and I baptized him before he died. He asked me if I would try to get the Catholic Church interested in the microbiological approach to psychiatry.

DR. EDWARD CARL ROSENOW, MAYO CLINIC

We got Dr. Rosenow to come down from Mayo, he worked out of Longview Hospital, and he isolated what he called the neurotropic streptococcus, which invades the central nervous system via the nasopharynx. By extracting the predominantly infecting virus or streptococcus from behind the nasopharynx, culturing it, and then injecting these in mice, pigs and rabbits, he produced the same symptoms as found in some mental patients. The animals all got

3

unprogrammed and confused. He tested 2,500+ patients at Longview Hospital and practically all were infected with the neurotropic streptococcus. Dr. Rosenow showed us that mental disorder can be caused by this virus, (see below reference) which is so small that one trillion can be contained in one cubic centimeter. They are also so strong, that they can live from 150 degrees below zero to 350 degrees above.

Dr. Rosenow tried to kill off this streptococcus by boiling them. He tried to make a thermal antibody by killing the virus and injecting it. You have to boil neurotrophic streptococcus for 96 hours to kill all of it. The streptococcus was boiled for 50 hours and put back into media and it started to grow again. He then boiled it in a 1.5% solution of <u>hydrogen peroxide</u> and killed off the streptococcus. Because of this phenomenon, I learned that there must be something really pertinent to using this strong potential killer of virus and streptococcus in the body.

REFERENCES

Subject. **"Bacteriologic, Etiologic, and Serologic Studies in Epilepsy and Schizophrenia III"**. May 1948 (Vol. 3, No. 5) issue of Postgraduate Medicine. Edward C. Rosenow, Longview Hospital Cincinnati, Ohio.

Subject: **"Influence of Streptococcal Infections on the Compulsive Behavior of Criminals."** Nov. 1951 (Vol 10, No. 5) Issue of Postgraduate Medicine. "Evidence that highly specific neurotropic toxins or poisons produced by a non-apparent type of streptococcal infection in nasopharynx or elsewhere may be responsible for the abnormal compulsions that characterize the behavior and acts of criminally inclined persons is reported."
- Edward C. Rosenow, Bacteriologic Research, Longview hospital, Cleveland, Ohio; Professor Emeritus, Experimental Bacteriology, Mayo Foundation, Rochester, Minnesota and O. F. Rosenow, Consulting Physician to the Ohio Penitentiary, Columbus, Ohio.

Subject: **"Bacteriological Studies in Idiopathic Epilepsy and Schizophrenia"** Address delivered by Dr. Rosenow to the South Dakota State Medical Association, Sioux Falls, South Dakota, May 20, 1952, and reprinted in the September, 1952, issue of the South Dakota Journal of Medicine and Pharmacy, Vol. V, No. 9, Pages 243-248; 262; 272. Paraphrased: Consistent isolation of these disease germs (alpha streptococci) in cases of idiopathic epilepsy and schizophrenia, and reproduction of the same disease symptoms in animals, and proof that there are specific membranes involved, indicate that persons suffering from epilepsy and from schizophrenia harbor, in the area of the throat behind the nose, or in pulpless teeth, or sometimes in their blood, specific types of alpha streptococci with neurotropic virulence, producing toxins that affect the brain. It is indicated that these germs and toxins may be affected by antigens and antibodies.

Subject: **"Studies on the nature of antibodies produced in vitro from bacteria with hydrogen peroxide and heat"**. Journal of Immunology, 55:219-232, 1947.

4

We now continue with Fr. Willhelm's narrative: After he retired, I went to see Dr. Rosenow at Mayo. He did basic research at Mayo for 62 years. (**Note: Dr. Rosenow 1875-1966, worked out the causes of some 35 different diseases and was the author of 450 medical papers. He was associated with the Mayo clinic for over 60 years. In 1914 he was considered America's most eminent bacteriologist. He discovered the streptococcus that caused Rheumatic Fever.**) Dr. Rosenow developed a technique by which microorganisms in the body could possibly be eliminated or controlled. The hydrogen peroxide program has resulted from his research. We know it as a method of taking oxygen into the body to eliminate or control these microorganisms. Rosenow suggested drinking hydrogen peroxide in a dilute solution. We've been preaching that gospel, drinking hydrogen peroxide. He also said take baths in it. I've been going about being a Catholic priest and you can't just jump into medicine, but my Bishop gave me permission to do that. I started a thing called "Educational Concern for Hydrogen Peroxide" (ECHO) and we've been trying to re-echo the voice, especially the voice of Our Lady of Lourdes.

OUR LADY OF LOURDES

We went to Lourdes in France, which is one of the most, probably the greatest shrine in all the world, and we tested Lourdes water. Lourdes water is loaded with hydrogen peroxide. The Blessed Virgin told someone from Lourdes to dig in the rock. A spring came up and she told her to drink the water and bathe in it. That's what the (hydrogen peroxide users) are trying to do. Dr. Donsbach is going one step further now. He is no longer bathing the outside of the body, but he is also bathing the bloodstream in it and he is getting tremendous results from it. We have, of course, a lot of opposition. You wonder why the medical establishment takes so long to come around and listen to this.

PHARMACEUTICAL HOUSE UNINTERESTED

We went to the headquarters of a large pharmaceutical firm. I told them about hydrogen peroxide and gave them my pamphlets. Their spokesperson said, "Father, I might as well be honest with you; You have to remember that we are a commercial venture. I can see no commercial value whatsoever in finding that hydrogen peroxide cures anything. You just can't make any money out of it." I guess that's why they've been holding up on it all these years. I finally got in touch with Dr. Charles H. Farr, who, along with Dr. Kurt Donsbach, is injecting hydrogen peroxide. We know there are a lot of doctors doing this throughout the country in their own small way. (Note: about 80-100). We hope that through the NHF we'll be able to convince our legislatures that this is a legitimate modality.

MENTAL ILLNESS

Father Schutte (had mental problems). Dr. Rosenow skin tested him. A big red blotch appeared where he tested him. He said that he had neurotropic streptococcus. He injected him with neurotropic streptococcus antibody from the hydrogen peroxide once a day.

After six weeks he went back to his prayers and hadn't had any recurrences since then. This eminent microbiologist maintained that mental illness can be caused by a neurotropic streptococcus.

Note: The cause might be the energy output of the microorganisms - the sending of confusing impulses into the nerve synapses.

EARTH'S OZONE

We have analyzed hydrogen peroxide. Hydrogen peroxide is H_2O_2. Water is H_2O. Hydrogen peroxide has an extra atom of nascent oxygen behind it. God, who made everything in the world, also gave us protection against things. Around the earth we have a big layer of oxygen. When the ultraviolet light from the sun comes down and hits this layer of oxygen around the earth, it turns oxygen (O_2) into O_3. It breaks up the one molecule atom and makes three atoms. This is ozone. Ozone is a bluish gas (that's why when we look up to the sky, the sky is blue during the day). There's a layer of ozone up there around the earth. That ozone; weighs more, and is heavier, than O_2 oxygen in the atmosphere, so it precipitates down through the atmosphere. When you bubble ozone through water, you turn water - H_2O, into H_2O_2 - hydrogen peroxide. Hydrogen peroxide comes down as rain. My mother used to put a pot out and collect rainwater to wash her hair and to water her flowers. What's the difference between rainwater and tap water? Test it yourself. Rainwater is loaded with hydrogen peroxide. You can water your grass all you want with tap water, it does a pretty good job. Just let it get rain! That grass picks up the hydrogen peroxide and the lawn turns green. All your fruits and vegetables have hydrogen peroxide. Note: W. Grotz has done retort tests to prove this, using the method listed in scientific encyclopedias.

Take one cubic inch of soil, it has between 100 thousand and 200 thousand bacteria in it. When the rain comes down it keeps down the bacteria in the soil and kills it off. By the time the water gets down to your deep well, it has lost all its hydrogen peroxide. A lot of the water in the lakes is full of hydrogen peroxide. The rain coming down has spent its hydrogen peroxide in oxidizing and making the pollution in the air non-toxic. We've lost a lot of the hydrogen peroxide in the process.

RAW FRUITS AND VEGETABLES

God looks after us. You've heard a lot about eating raw fruits and vegetables. You've heard Charlotte Gerson; her therapy is giving you an 8 oz. glass of freshly squeezed vegetable juice, orange juice or liver juice every hour on the hour. She doesn't tell you the reason why these things are good for you; why they have to be raw, why they have to be crushed and squeezed. It's because all your fruits and vegetables have collected that hydrogen peroxide coming down in the rain. It's stored in fruits and vegetables. When you eat them raw, you get the hydrogen peroxide. Man is the only animal that has processed his food. All other animals eat it raw. They eat the seeds too. In processing our food we have lost this very important substance.

Note: Furton & Simmonds's "General Biochemistry", p.338 states that
hydrogen peroxide in fruits and vegetables is true. If we were to
eat uncooked fresh fruit and vegetables, we would get more oxygen
in our bodies. Is this why so many vegetable, fruit, etc., diets
are so popular and widely claimed to be effective in curing all
sorts of so-called "incurable" diseases?

THERE WAS NO CANCER IN THE SEA FULL OF TRACE MINERALS AND H_2O_2

I worked with Dr. Murray. Murray was a captain of the sea.
He found out there was no cancer in the sea (this was over 25 years
ago and assumes an unpolluted, naturally clean sea). He dissected
964 whales. He kept track of them. In the sea all the mammals and
fish were cancer free. They had none of the systemic diseases.
Most fish die by getting eaten up by bigger ones. The shark
usually dies in battle. Dr. Murray tested the water in the sea.
The water in the sea contains all of the trace elements. We
located a deposit of sea salt down in the Baja Peninsula near San
Philipe and Mexicali. They have a rich deposit of sea salt there.
He wrote a book about sea energy agriculture, getting the elements
out of the sea back into the soil. All the "goodies" have been
washed off with our soil, and are out there in the sea. The sea
elements are great. Dr. Murray never tested sea water for hydrogen
peroxide. Sea water is loaded with hydrogen peroxide. That's why
his fish ware free of disease, because the fish were living in a
sea of hydrogen peroxide. (16) Ponce De Leon was looking for the
fountain of youth... There it was; right in the sea!

Note: The pollution in the seas is presently reaching such levels,
that with the oceanic oxygen levels dropping off, even the seals in
Norway are dieing of viral diseases.

Hydrogen peroxide--you can buy 3% solution in the drugstore or
your grocery store. It isn't even a drug. You scrub your teeth
with baking soda and sea salt, or salt, and rinse your mouth with
hydrogen peroxide it gets rid of gum disease. If you put hydrogen
peroxide on healthy skin, nothing much happens. If you put
hydrogen peroxide on a sore, or where you have infection, it
bubbles up and it gives off oxygen and kills all the bacteria.
Hydrogen peroxide was made by God and it's a very important factor
in keeping down the bacteria throughout the world.

Note: April 12, 1913, 75 years ago, Mr. Seward told the Southern
Counties Branch of the British Dental Association he had hit upon
a very satisfactory treatment for removing tartar, the underlying
cause of pyorrhea, by the use of a dentifrice containing perborate
of soda, which in the presence of organic matter splits up with the
formation of hydrogen peroxide, which again splits up into water
and nascent oxygen.

An interesting thing; If you test sea water with a solution
of ferrous sulfate and potassium iodine, it gives off the iodine
and the water turns yellow. This yellow color proves the presence
of peroxide. Using the same test, we find that sea salt is loaded
with hydrogen peroxide. When it comes down in the rain it goes
into the sea, you don't have as many bacteria in the sea as you
have in the soil. The sea maintains its hydrogen peroxide. When
you boil low concentrations of hydrogen peroxide you don't break it

7

up. (Note: Walter has boiled it and tested the remainder, and it still tests positive with the potassium iodide test. In a weak solution, hydrogen peroxide is distillable with water) It goes up in steam, you condense it back down into water and the water (you end up with) is about the same strength as (the water you started with) before you boil it. You don't destroy hydrogen peroxide by boiling it. That's a very important thing. When the water evaporates from the sea, it brings up the hydrogen peroxide and it rains it back down on the earth. You have a complete cycle.

ELECTRICAL STORMS PRODUCE H_2O_2

According to the AMA Journal, printed March 30th, of 1888 - and reprinted in 1988 - During a lightning storm, the high potential electricity produces hydrogen peroxide. If you get high potential electricity and put oxygen over it, it turns the oxygen into ozone. I made an ozone machine for Dr. Murray 42 years ago. I wired some electrodes that caused a big spark, an old transformer (from a beer sign) and put 15,000 volts to it, pumped oxygen through the can I put it in, and ozone came out the other side. 40 years ago Dr. Murray and I bubbled ozone through blood. It turned some diseased blood which was kind of dark & brownish, into real light red, then we injected it back into the patient. A doctor that I was working with from Dusseldorf, Germany is doing the same treatment today, 40 years later! Ozone is a very important thing. Also, hydrogen peroxide. Hydrogen peroxide and ozone are compatible because when you bubble ozone through water, it turns water (H_2O) into H_2O_2, by adding O_1.

MILK

Dr. Rosenow - and how he was a great doctor. In Minneapolis there was a polio epidemic in one of the high schools. Rosenow went there and found the polio virus in the milk they were drinking. "Your milk is loaded with bacteria". Dr. Murray didn't keep a drop of milk in his house for 45 years. He said: "You see how it is. There is bacteria in it, that's why it sours". Those little bugs in there start to multiply and the milk sours. If you put a teaspoonful of hydrogen peroxide (3% that you buy in the store) in a quart of milk, the milk will never sour. All around the world they are using hydrogen peroxide in milk. They've been doing it for 25 years in Russia, and Korea. As soon as they milk the cow, they put hydrogen peroxide in it. They do it in their own kitchens. There are a lot of people who won't drink milk unless it is treated with hydrogen peroxide. We found that the hydrogen peroxide that you can buy in the store is fine.

PATENT OFFICE HAS METHODS OF H_2O_2 CREATION

I went to the U.S. Patent Office in Washington. They have about 25 different ways to make hydrogen peroxide. Some of the hydrogen peroxide you get in the store tastes a little different because they put in stabilizers. We found out there is a food grade hydrogen peroxide available.

FOOD GRADE USED IN WINE & CHEESE WORLDWIDE

Food Grade H_2O_2 is used in milk all over the world. Carlo Rossi (the winemaker) says he puts hydrogen peroxide in the wine to bleach the wine. It is used for making cheese. Hydrogen peroxide is the most beneficial thing you can drink. You have to take it in the proper proportion. We have available 35% hydrogen peroxide that is food quality.

We found out that when you drink hydrogen peroxide it goes into your stomach and in 13 seconds it will be out at the end of your fingers. We can also drink radioactive iodine and in 13 seconds the radioactivity is out at the end of your finger. Hydrogen peroxide breaks up, but not until it comes in contact with virus and streptococcus.   - End of Fr. Willhelm's talk.

FURTHER INFORMATION

In further conversations with Father Willhelm, I discovered that the best way to find out about this subject is to go to the Mayo clinic and read Dr. Rosenow's papers. Dr. Rosenow even went to the point, in his research, that he was performing experiments that showed streptococcus mutating by exposure to normal cosmic radiation.

One of the latest health fads is "Live Cell Therapy". 45 years ago, Fr. Willhelm and Dr. Murray were taking cells from the thymus gland of unborn calves, and injecting it into patients. The thymus gland regulates the production of antibodies so an infant doesn't reject it's mother's organs. After birth, we develop our own antibodies. The injection of these cells is supposed to stimulate antibody production in humans.

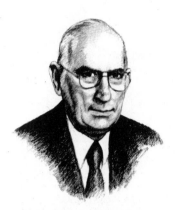

WALTER GROTZ

THE FOREMOST HYDROGEN PEROXIDE PROPONENT IN THE U.S.

WALTER GROTZ ACCEPTS PIONEER AWARD

MC at award presentation: "Walter Grotz became interested in the hydrogen peroxide story after meeting Father Willhelm. Walter had a number of health problems which disappeared after he used hydrogen peroxide and he is here to excite us with this amazing product."

From here on, Walter Grotz is speaking, assume quotes:

There is a true saying that behind every man there is a great woman. Our case is not an exception. Ladies and gentlemen, if it was not for my bride of almost 40 years, I would not be here today. Because it was at her insistence that I go on this Caribbean cruise where I met Father Willhelm. Ladies and gentlemen, our lives have not been the same since. I would like you people to meet this Mary Grotz of mine and give her a round of applause.

Now, I did say our case was not an exception. The lady behind Father Willhelm, that he proudly displays on the front of his literature. Her name is also Mary. It was Father Willhelm that kept this little spark alive for many years, even though behind the scenes much research was going on.

For many years the average person thought that hydrogen peroxide had but one use. The FDA had that same idea, even up until June 13, 1985 in the Washington Post. 'Hydrogen peroxide is only good for bleaching hair.'

Father Willhelm has been ridiculed. He has been opposed; even by his own family. I've been with his friends. They say that Father Dick is one heck of a great guy, but there is this peroxide thing...

10

Dr. Edward Carl Rosenow; I'm certain he was a great inspiration to Father Willhelm and also to myself. He used hydrogen peroxide to prepare his antibodies.

Dr. Oliver, in 1919, had the courage to inject hydrogen peroxide intravenously. He wrote about it in the Lancet so that we had record of it. Dr. Otto Warburg, twice Nobel Laureate, talked about how a cancer cell was a fermenting cell, and a healthy cell was an oxidizing cell. He went so far as to prove that cancer cannot grow in a high oxygen environment.(9)

Note: Dr. Warburg won the Nobel Prize in Medicine, in 1931, for his discovery of the oxygen transferring enzyme of cell respiration. He won a second Nobel Prize, in 1944, for his discovery of the active groups of the hydrogen transferring enzymes.

Dr. William Frederick Koch, when I hear his name I want to hang my head in shame; (what the establishment did to that man!) I had the privilege of spending five hours with the man who was with Dr. Koch when he died. He used a substance called glyoxylide. OXY right in the center; oxygen. He spoke about how the oxygen in glyoxylide was the same oxygen that was in hydrogen peroxide. In his book, in 1926, he said yes, people who have cancer were to drink hydrogen peroxide. So we hear of Hydrogen peroxide's use way back in 1926!

Robert Stroud ("The Birdman of Alcatraz") spent over 50 years in solitary confinement. He healed little birds using hydrogen peroxide and sodium perborate. Sodium perborate in water gives you hydrogen peroxide. That's how he got the name, "The Birdman of Alcatraz".

Dr. Reginald Holeman, at the St. Thomas Laboratory in Cardiff, Wales, in the middle 50's, gave cancerous mice .3% hydrogen peroxide in their drinking water, and in 60 days the cancerous tumors disappeared. Hydrogen peroxide gained a little bit of merit in the treatment of cancer.

Winifred Wirth, a little slip of a lady, fought cancer many times herself. In 1982 and 1983, she gave cancerous mice hydrogen peroxide. (15) (16) All she did was reconfirm the work done by Dr. Reginald Holeman from Cardiff, Wales. Clinton Miller, who heard us speak in Washington, DC, told me: "This message must get out to the American people." I hear it was Clinton Miller who convinced Hal Card, Maureen Sullivan, & Dr. Donsbach, to give me the opportunity to bring this word throughout our nation. George Borell, who just wrote the book, "The Peroxide Story"; Betsy Manning had enough courage to write a chapter in her book. All of these people, I'm giving credit to, as I accept the Pioneer Award. Thank You.

WALTER GROTZ SPEAKS TO MINNESOTA INSTITUTE OF HEALTH

It is indeed a pleasure for me to be here, and I appreciate the opportunity to speak to the Minnesota Institute of Health. Two years ago I didn't even know the hydrogen peroxide program existed. In these past two years, I have learned a tremendous number of things.

WALTER GROTZ FIRST LEARNS OF PEROXIDE

I became interested in this program under rather unusual circumstances. I met a retired Army chaplain, Father Richard Willhelm. He told me that he had dedicated the remainder of his life to furthering the work of Dr. Edward Carl Rosenow, which meant nothing to me. I am sure it doesn't mean anything to a lot of you people too. He told me that this doctor had over 450 published medical papers. He spent over 60 years doing basic research with the Mayo Clinic. His research papers are filed in the library of the Mayo Clinic.

WE LIVE IN AN OCEAN OF MICROORGANISMS

In 1925, Dr. Rosenow discovered that rheumatic fever was caused by a streptococcus germ. His basic tenet was that we live in an ocean of microorganisms, and that our body is like a world. In the world of the body are millions of microorganisms; each little creature, depending upon what kind it is, seeks out it's own individual area or environment to feed on and grow in. These microorganisms can give you dandruff. They live in your hair, and in your mouth. They can give you cavities and all kinds of mouth diseases. Way down to your feet, they can give you athlete's foot, and they will set up housekeeping in all regions in between.

Note: I will interrupt for a moment to insert this chart of what Mr. Grotz's E.C.H.O. Newsletter has to say about these anaerobic, can't live in oxygen, microorganisms. These "bugs", or, microorganisms, do the following:

-gnaw away at the joints (inflammatory arthritis)
-give off calcium waste-matter that cements bones together
-lodge in liver and kidneys, and with their bile, form stones
-live in the very lining of the arteries, and leave their hard deposit on the walls of the arteries (arterial plaque)
-cling to the lining in the nervous system and short-circuit some of the electronics in the central computer of the brain
-attack cells and enter them, building cocoons around the stricken cell; thus cutting off the blood supply and causing the cell to lose its specific function, so that it can only live and multiply into cancerous tumors

Now back to the narrative.

I listened to this retired Army chaplain and he also told me that there was a program how we could possibly control or eliminate these microorganisms from our body. He told me that the program was drinking a simple solution of hydrogen peroxide.

With my limited amount of chemistry, I could see the possibility of this working. I had arthritis in my right elbow and in my knees and in my left ankle. Walking was painful. My knee was painful to the touch. What did I have to lose? I started through the program. After one week it caused me to vomit. I called up Father Willhelm and I said, "Hey, your stuff made me vomit! I don't like to vomit, it makes me sick!" He said, "Vomiting is a very natural thing. Pregnant women do it all the time." (Note: Most people don't vomit on peroxide, but at the same time, many people do get some nauseous sensations from it.) That was my sympathy. Two days later, I was back on the program. In 16 days I started noticing relief.

Then came the big thing. I had to know why and how. There were some questions I had to have answered. The only way that I could possibly get them answered was to get into this thing 24 hours a day and seven days a week. The questions were these: 1) Was it quackery? 2) Was it just psychosomatic? 3) Was this stuff natural? 4) Could there possibly be a scientific approach? Let's take the first one; quackery.

QUACKERY?

I called up a Cancer Information Service, an 800 number, because I wanted to get updated on a certain cancer cure. In the course of the conversation, the woman said that this was quackery. I said, "What's quackery? "Is quackery something that costs a lot of money and doesn't do any good?" She said, "That is the best explanation I've heard." Do you know how much it cost me to get rid of my arthritis? Less than $6.00! If it is quackery, I'll guarantee you this; the price is right!

PSYCHOSOMATIC? (IS IT ALL IN THE MIND?)

Was it psychosomatic? A man told me that he heard this on the radio; (the Dick Pomerantz show, on April 30, 1982.) He told his wife, because he had arthritis, "I know this isn't going to work, but, I'm going to try it." I think that man is here today. Even with his negative attitude it worked. So that kind of ruled out the psychosomatic thing. What could this thing be?

NATURAL OR POISON?

Natural? So, I went to people who I thought could give me the proper answers. Natural? Heck, no! That stuff is poison! What's poison about it? What's it made out of? Well, it's made out of water. Is water poison? No. But it has oxygen in it. Is oxygen poison? It better not be, or we'd all be dead! Hydrogen peroxide is H_2O_2. It is water plus another oxygen. (H_2O is water, O is oxygen. $H_2O + O = H_2O_2$.) That's all it is.

Note for scientists: Granted, some natural substances can be hazardous if we add a single atom to them, but this doesn't seem to be the case here. Concentration is a strong determining factor.

ASKS DOCTORS

The doctor told me that in medical school, all they ever told him about hydrogen peroxide is that it bubbled and killed germs. If it kills germs it should have interested somebody! (3) Another one told me that hydrogen peroxide doesn't kill anything, all it does is bubble. I said, "Doctor, what's an antiseptic?" He cursed me over the telephone. I said, "Doctor, not over the telephone." He hung up.

LIBRARY SEARCH SHOWS PEROXIDE IN RAIN & SNOW

Where am I to go for information? I turned to our libraries, the first time in my life I ever used libraries, and I cannot say enough for librarians. They bent over backwards to help me. One of the first things they came up with was out of McGraw Hill's Encyclopedia of Science, the Fifth Edition, p. 728; that hydrogen peroxide exists in rain and snow. How does it get there? I do not believe that God does things just for the sake of doing things. I think He's got other things to do. There must be a reason. How does it get there? From the ozone layer. I'm sure you've read and heard enough that the environmentalists are all worried that we're going to destroy the ozone layer.

SUNSHINE FORMS OZONE DAILY

How does the ozone layer get there? From the sunlight, where all the energy for life comes from. The sun. It is the ultraviolet light. The shorter the blues, the longer the violets are, 185 millimeters long. The ultraviolet light splits the free oxygen O_2, the molecule of oxygen containing two atoms. The two oxygen atoms are held together by a covalent bond. Because the single atom of oxygen is short two electrons on its outer orbit, it has to share with another atom of oxygen. The sun's ultraviolet light splits the bond. Now this newly formed atom of two oxygens (O_2) hooks onto another molecule of oxygen (O_1), giving you ozone, which is O_3.

OZONE CREATES HYDROGEN PEROXIDE IN RAIN

Now ozone is heavier than oxygen, so it starts settling down. Our high flying jet airplanes are having a problem with it. They fly into clouds of it. It gets into their fresh air intakes. Through their air exchangers, It gets into the cabin. It irritates the lungs of the passengers. This is documented in medical books. It keeps settling down. As soon as it touches the moisture, (water) it turns into hydrogen peroxide. It gets into our rain. If it is not destroyed by pollution, it reaches the ground. It gets into our fruits and vegetables. Also, it is manufactured in the photosynthesis process of plants, and we get it into our systems. Man is the only creature on earth that processes his food before he eats it. But, he also processes it for his animals. So we have veterinarians to take care of animals. We are what we eat and our animals are what we feed them.

W. GROTZ FINDS HEALTH MEETINGS

I started to go to my first health meeting with this group listening to Dr. Mendelsohn. That was on March 25, 1982. I didn't even know these people existed. Then I started going to health conventions. I listened to Charlotte Gerson. I listened to Edie May, I listened to Ann Wigmore. I was convinced that their therapies worked. I knew that the one I went through worked. I got to thinking, there must be a correlation between the two. There must be a common denominator. What is that missing link?

GROTZ PEROXIDE EXPERIMENTS

So I went back home and I took my wife's kitchen utensils and I turned her kitchen into a laboratory. I started cooking and brewing. The first thing I found out was that hydrogen peroxide is not as unstable as they say it is. They say you've got to store it lower than 90 degrees. No way. You can take 3% and you can boil it and you cannot liberate enough oxygen to re-ignite the glowing split, the test for oxygen. Let it cool down, put some potassium iodide in it, you've got all kinds of oxygen. I kept on going, and I accidentally got a theory. With this theory I checked the hydrogen peroxide content in raw fruits and vegetables.

Note: Whenever Mr. Grotz refers to something having peroxide in it, it is because he has tested it with the chemical encyclopedia test using potassium iodide and ferrous sulfate that will test down to one part of hydrogen peroxide to twenty million parts of water.

Note: Some supermarkets in California are misting their fresh fruits and vegetables with hydrogen peroxide. They find it increases the shelf life. Could this replace nitrites used in restaurants and food preserving?

PEROXIDE IN MOTHERS MILK

With this test, I checked the hydrogen peroxide content in milk. Unpasteurized milk has more than pasteurized milk. So twice we checked and analyzed human mother's milk to find out that it contained a high percentage of hydrogen peroxide. Now don't tell me you can find anything more natural than that.

COLOSTRUM MILKS

Then we got into the colostrum milks. Colostrum milk, according to the dictionary, is the first milk secreted after birth containing high amounts of protein and immunizing factors for the newborn, because mammals are born without antibodies. We have tested it and found that it contains a higher amount of hydrogen peroxide than regular milk. Very much higher.

Note: There is a great alternative health interest, recently, in drinking colostrum milk. Could it's effects be from the peroxide?

15

IS VITAMIN "U" PEROXIDE?

How many of you people have heard of vitamin U? Very few people have. If you want to learn more about it, go to the medical library. The work was done in the 1940's by Dr. Garnet Chaney in San Francisco. (19) He found it in unpasteurized milk. He found it in the fresh fruits and vegetables. He found a high amount in cabbage. He found it in the yolk of the egg, exactly where we find the hydrogen peroxide. It tracks vitamin U to the letter. He used cabbage juice to cure ulcers. He gave them one quart of cabbage juice each day, and in 16 days their ulcers were gone.

SCIENCE TESTS PEROXIDE

So then, the scientific approach. In Cardiff, Wales, a doctor gave cancerous mice hydrogen peroxide in their drinking water and found that the tumors went into remission. This is also documented in the medical library. We had this experiment duplicated in Cincinnati, Ohio, in Dr. Sperti's cancer lab (15). Who is this Dr. Sperti? He holds 23 medical patents. The Sperti Sunlamp is his. How about Preparation H? That is his. Aspergum is his. They did 14 months of research for us. 80% cleaning up of the cancerous mice is no problem. In May of 1983 when they wound it up, they had 90%. (16)

PEROXIDE ULTIMATE CAUSE OF CELL DIVISION?

Somebody in the United States sent me what looked like the front page of a medical article. It was done in the University of Iowa, University of Wisconsin, and Wabash College, Crawfordsville, Indiana. In the bottom of the last paragraph were these words: "We hypothesize", which means we have looked at the facts, this is our conclusion; "we hypothesize that hydrogen peroxide is the ultimate cause of normal cell division." Normal cell division. (5)

I called this doctor and talked to him. He said that since we did that, we have taken the hydrogen peroxide away from the livers of hamsters and the liver cells immediately turned into fetal cells, or tumor cells. (Note: See also, the section on cell mutation, under Rife Microscopes.) I went to Iowa City, where the doctor lives, and talked to him for three hours. I turned tapes and data on hydrogen peroxide over to him. He sent me a letter and called me on the telephone. He said, "I believe you guys have got it." I said, "Look, doctor, I only think in simple terms." He said, "That's the problem, it's so simple we went right over the top."

There's a debate going on now. Who's going to get credit? I wouldn't give any present day scientist credit. Mine goes back to 1910 to Dr. William Frederick Koch. Everytime I hear his name I'm not too proud to be an American. We put him through three trials. Three trials by the American Medical Association and the FDA. We exiled that man to Brazil where he died in 1968. Note: See section on Koch.

MEDICAL RESEARCH

So they got anxious about getting into doing research. They are doing research right now for us. They started the last week in June and the results that are coming out of there are absolutely exciting. Everything is controlled. Everything is done on the scientific basis.

COMPUTER SEARCH

We did a computer search on the medical library. We put in human blood and hydrogen peroxide. Were we surprised! 33 articles came up. Then we got into the Index Medicus. There are over 1,000 published articles on hydrogen peroxide. In 1983 there will be over 100 medical articles done on it.

PEROXIDE KILLS BACTERIA

Here is another article: "Hydrogen Peroxide, The Medicated Killing of Bacteria". Leukocytes have multiple systems available for killing ingested bacteria that we either breathe in or swallow. Nearly each of these incorporate hydrogen peroxide - indicating the essential nature of this reactive oxygen.

LACK OF PEROXIDE OPENS WAY FOR INFECTION

Now in the same article: "These mechanisms appear important, since deficiencies of hydrogen peroxide production and lactoferrin frequently increase the owner's susceptibility to infection."(17)

PEROXIDE IN BLOOD

Hydrogen peroxide is released from human blood platelets. (4) (21) Now, as we know, human blood platelets are used in the treatment of leukemia. How about the removal of cholesterol and other lipids (type of fatty deposit) from experimental animal and human arteries by dilutants of hydrogen peroxide? (6)

VIRUS CAUSES HARD ARTERIES?

They took hardened arteries that were so hard you could snap them like macaroni, they soaked them in hydrogen peroxide, and they became soft. Within the last couple of weeks, it was in the St. Paul paper, it said that hardening of the arteries is caused by a virus similar to herpes.

CELLS PRODUCE H_2O_2

There was an article that was done in India. The generation of hydrogen peroxide in the biomembranes. (7) We are getting right down into the cells. It says: "The generation of hydrogen peroxide in cellular processes seems to be purposeful and hydrogen peroxide cannot be dismissed as a mere undesirable by-product."

INTERFERON AND PEROXIDE

How many people here have heard of interferon? They say it is supposed to be the wonder drug of the century. This comes from The Journal of Interferon Research. The results suggest that interferon may stimulate the production of low amounts of hydrogen peroxide. "We present evidence here which is compatible with the suggestion that hydrogen peroxide and possible other oxygen intermediates play a role in the function of the cells", which they call the NK cell, it's a natural killer cell. Also, "these results raise the possibility that the response generated by interferon may be due to the liberation of hydrogen peroxide."(2)

GERSON

Charlotte Gerson (Has a clinic that specializes in the Gerson therapy), in one of her lectures said that: "We do not take people who have had transplants, because we activate the immune system to the point where rejection takes place."

TRANSPLANTS

I went through the journals of transplants and ran into it in the Journal of Transplantation, July, 1983. (20) It talks about the problem that the hydrogen peroxide that is generated by the body attacks the implant. What they have to do is give something to suppress it. When they do, they suppress the immune system. What happened to the last liver transplant? It was a success. He died of the flu. He had no immune system left.

PEROXIDE VITAL TO IMMUNE SYSTEM

It is my firm belief that hydrogen peroxide is part of the immune system of the body. I gave a talk in Chicago June 25, and Charlotte Gerson heard me. She went back to California and went through the program, as did Norman Fritz. Norman had an immediate flare up of his malaria, which he thinks will be gone from now on.

Note: Initial "cleansing reactions" - that mimic all the symptoms of past illnesses, in reverse order - are commonly reported in the early stages of peroxide therapies.

MALARIA

One more article here. Malaria. This article was done in January 1983. The killing of blood stage "murine", which means mouse, malaria parasites by hydrogen peroxide. (8)

LANCET MEDICAL JOURNAL

The Lancet is the most prestigious medical journal in the world. It will stand up to the New England Journal of Medicine. A February 12, 1983 article described how this free radical kills malaria. Another article in the February Lancet indicated that oxygen will destroy malaria. But they've got a debate on over who is going to get credit.

They're debating who's going to get credit, when in 1984, 200 million people in the world will contract malaria. I wouldn't give either one of those guys credit for it. Mine goes back to Dr. Koch in 1910.

FLU STOPPED BY PEROXIDE IN 1920

There was an article in the Lancet February 21, 1920, when the big flu epidemic was going around the world. In a hospital in India, 80% of the people in one ward were dying from influenzal pneumonia. Nothing worked. They took the worst patient they had in the hospital, who was delirious for two days. He had to be tied in bed owing to his delirium. They took two ounces of hydrogen peroxide at 3%, mixed it with eight ounces of saline solution. It tells how they injected him. In six hours the man was sitting up and asking for food.

1884 ORAL USAGE OF PEROXIDE

If you want to get into the oral use of hydrogen peroxide, that's a whole new ball game. The oldest article we have is 1884. Hydrogen peroxide has been on the market for a long time as an over-the-counter drug; if you want to call it a drug. I was looking through the Physician's Desk Reference and I can't find it in there.

PEROXIDE TWICE AS OLD AS ASPIRIN

Hydrogen peroxide was first reported in 1818 by a French chemist, Louis-Jaques Thenard, who called it, "eau oxygenee". That's how old it is. It's twice as old as aspirin. It is so simple.

MANY USES FOR H_2O_2

Hydrogen peroxide has been used for many things. In World War II Adolf Hitler powered his V-2 rockets with it. In Cape Canaveral they use it as an oxygen source. The most common strength we know is 3%. Then you can get some 6% that the girls put in their hair.

H_2O_2 USED IN FOOD

Hydrogen peroxide is used in food products. It is called food-grade hydrogen peroxide. If you go to a pharmacist and ask him for food-grade peroxide, he will probably shake his head and say there is no such thing. On January 9, 1981, the FDA gave the green light to the food industry to use food grade hydrogen peroxide for aseptic packaging.

H_2O_2 USED TO PRESERVE MILK AND FRUIT JUICE

These are long shelf life milk cartons (Shows samples). They come from California and Savannah, Georgia. They use it to put milk on the shelf for up to eight months without refrigeration. It's called the aseptic package. They are the little juice boxes where you jab the straw in the top. They use hydrogen peroxide. There is a good article on aseptic packaging in Trailer Life magazine, February 1981.

Note: The Food & Drug Administration issued Federal Regulation Vol. 46, Number 6, on January 9, 1981 for the hydrogen peroxide "Aseptic" process.

Do you think anybody would drink the juice if they knew there was hydrogen peroxide in there? No way, because they've been told it's poison.

H_2O_2 IN CONTACT LENS CLEANERS & EYE DROPS

Here are some hydrogen peroxide products: Lensept. If you've got contact lenses, after a couple of years you can't wear them anymore. You go back to the man that sold them to you. He says after a couple of years your body will reject the contact lenses. Somebody figured out why. It appears as though microorganisms get into the plastic and irritate your eyes. So you soak them overnight in Lensept.

Then we have Murine, which is a peroxide for cleaning your ears. And Oxy 10, which is for acne. It's 10% hydrogen peroxide.

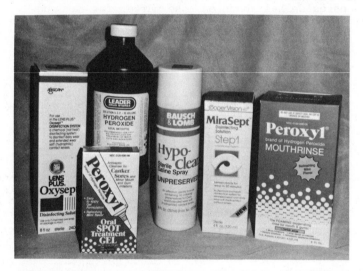

COMMON DRUGSTORE PRODUCTS CONTAINING PEROXIDE

CATALYST ALTERED WATERS

Then, we have catalyst altered waters. There are over 100 companies making these now. Willard Water was analyzed by the FDA and they said that all it was, was distilled water plus the additives on the outside. I took one taste of it, and the people here that have drank hydrogen peroxide will agree with me, once you've tasted it you'll never forget it. Taste does not tell me anything. It has to be done scientifically. So I took the sample over to the Twin City Testing Company in St. Paul. It cost me $100 to verify the fact; a certified test showed it contained hydrogen peroxide. The catalyst people claim the difference is that the electrons are spinning in the opposite direction from their spins in hydrogen peroxide.

FDA REQUIRES MOUTHWASHES TO HAVE H_2O_2

We have a thing called Medident. In the FDA regulations it says that mouthwashes should have hydrogen peroxide in them. We tested it. Yes, it does have hydrogen peroxide.

H_2O_2 IN ALOE VERA

Aloe vera, you know, the plant you use when you have a burn or sunburn. Now they have an aloe vera juice, and when people drink it, they say it tastes like peroxide. They say aloe vera juice tastes like peroxide. They are right. It has it in there naturally because of the photosynthesis process.

H_2O_2 IN LAETRILE

There is hydrogen peroxide in laetrile. We put it through the test, and a high amount of oxygen, not necessarily always hung up with hydrogen peroxide, shows up. It can be in other peroxides and other "ides". They say that laetrile is nothing but cyanide. Our tests show we are bringing out this atomic radical oxygen in the test. That single O.

KOCH GLYOXYLIDE

Dr. Koch's Glyoxylide, which I got a ruling from the FDA, it's called, "Cancer Quackery, Past and Present." It says Dr. Koch's Glyoxylide was nothing but distilled water. We went to the FDA in Rockville, Maryland, and we talked to the people who did the work on Willard Water, and we asked them, "Did you test it for hydrogen peroxide?" They said "We never did and we never will." In fact, the man actually said, "We don't know how." We left the test for them. In Dr. Koch's Glyoxylide, it shows up very strong. Dr. Koch talks about the oxidation reduction mechanism. Note: Please refer to the section on Dr. Koch.

DMSO - CLOROX

Then we have DMSO. The O is the oxygen. Again, you have the "oxide" on the end. The Clorox. It's a super oxide. If you start studying it chemically as a bleach, they say that the oxygen is the one that's doing the bleaching. Oxygen is at the bottom of many reactions.

BIRDMAN OF ALCATRAZ

Then we get into sodium perborate. Sodium perborate in water gives you hydrogen peroxide. When I was in Chicago, a lady came out of the audience and said "Did you read the book The Birdman of Alcatraz? (Robert Stroud was a famous prisoner who kept birds and wrote books on their care.) Do you know what he used to cure those birds?" He used sodium perborate in water which gives hydrogen peroxide. The Birdman of Alcatraz! Fifty years ago!

CHICKENS

In Pennsylvania we have flocks of chickens drinking hydrogen peroxide because of the Avian flu, which has broken out in Lancaster County and in the neighboring states, and it is not just confined to chickens, but it's also into the turkeys. They have had to destroy 9 million chickens in an attempt to stop it's spread. "Birdman" Stroud said that 50 years down the road, sodium perborate and hydrogen peroxide will come into their own. That was in 1939. We're almost there. Stroud spent 54 years in solitary confinement. It's a very interesting book.

H_2O_2 IN WATER

We went to Europe and checked a lot of the waters. I could taste hydrogen peroxide in the Greek water. They say it's natural. But in Europe they use ozone and hydrogen peroxide in a lot of their city waters instead of chlorine, because ozone has 5,000 times the killing power over chlorine on bacteria. (Note: See sections on industrial, municipal, and spa and pool uses of ozone.) It's in Perrier water. The naturally carbonated water from France gets it's carbonation and traces of hydrogen peroxide from bubbling up from deep in the earth.

H_2O_2 IN COMMERCIAL AIRLINE WATER

Flying over to Europe on a TWA airplane, I could taste hydrogen peroxide in their water. My companions said, "You've got peroxide on the brain." I got out my test kit and tested it. I went to the stewardess. I asked what's wrong with your water? She said that there could be nothing wrong with the water. The plane just came out of maintenance in New York, and they just flushed the tanks out with hydrogen peroxide.

HEALING SPRINGS

We went to Lourdes. We went to the medical bureau. When we came in the door, the secretary said, to Fr. Willhelm, "I know you! You're the Peroxide Priest!" She asked, "What do you want here?" I said that we were going to test the water for hydrogen peroxide. She wanted to know why we wanted to do that. She said that Sloane Kittering was there several times and they tested it for everything and found it was pure water. I asked if they tested it for hydrogen peroxide. She said no.

This is St. Ann's water from Quebec, Canada. There's a spring there. This is water from Kidney Hot Springs in Hot Springs, South Dakota. The Indians used to fight battles over who had control of these springs. It was a health resort. The Evans plunge is still there yet. It is almost a ghost town. It has a high amount of hydrogen peroxide in it naturally.

Highway 18 has a spring that's south of Eden Prairie, Minnesota. Very good water. Soap Lake, Washington. It was on TV twice. It's a place where all the water comes down the mountains and is collected into one lake. People go in there and bathe in it and they drink it. If you think hydrogen peroxide is bad to drink, try some of that! It also has some salt in it.

RAIN

Rainwater. You'll get different amounts of concentrations depending on what kind of rainstorm you have. If there is a lot of lightning, you'll get more hydrogen peroxide. Says so in the encyclopedias.

Note: A friend of the family told me about her father brewing some "Bathtub Gin", during Prohibition. Seems that if there was a lightning storm, the fermentation would stop completely, and he'd have to start over. Lightning storms produce ozone in the air that also turns into H_2O_2. This high level of ozone in the atmosphere, which stops alcohol from brewing, makes a good analogy. Fermentation is an anaerobic process. It is the same as the action of having a high oxygen level in the body halting the lives of most disease bacteria, viruses, and other pathogens, which all rely upon a fermentation (or without oxygen) way of "breathing".

FOODS

We checked raw comb honey and found there is hydrogen peroxide in it. Some say that it's a by-product. I say the honey bee puts it in there as a preservative. The raw eggs. You'll see that the yolk has more peroxide in it than the white of the egg. Then we got into checking the aseptic "long shelf life" milk. If you test it, you'll see that it contains some. Next we tested livers; calf liver, pork liver, and lake trout liver. We found they contain hydrogen peroxide. Now we know why, when you go to Charlotte Gerson's clinic, you have to drink that 8 ounces of emulsified raw calf's liver twice a day. Then we get into raw milks. You have it in the human mother's milk, goat's milk, cow's milk, the cow's colostrum & blood. We didn't test any human blood. How about sprouts? When the sprouts start to sprout, the vitamins go up and the hydrogen peroxide level also goes up.

PENICILLIN

Penicillin. What's a reason it works so well? A medical paper says: "The oxidation of glucose by O2 in the presence of penicillin, results in the formation of bactericidal amounts of hydrogen peroxide."(1)

SUPER OXIDE DISMUTASE

Super oxide dismutase. It turns into a hydrogen peroxide. You'll find that a lot in medical articles. They talk about the super oxide dismutase you can buy it in pills. A research doctor in Iowa said that the best is made from young calf's liver. Back to the calf's liver again. Note: See special section on high potency, wheat grass Super Oxide Dismutase.

ORANGE JUICE

Now these are the vegetables. Fresh orange juice. A Doctor talked to this group sometime ago and in this tape or lecture he said that if a physician sends a patient to the hospital and prescribes orange juice, that patient should get fresh squeezed orange juice and not reconstituted from a can. So we went to talk to him in Chicago for two and a half hours, asking him, "Why, doctor?" He said if you use your city water with your chlorine and your fluorine in it to make the juice.... I said, yes, I'll agree with you. I said, what if they used distilled water? He said there would be a difference. I asked what the difference would be. He finally said he didn't know. Within 48 hours we knew. We put it through an analyzer. Freshly squeezed juice has hydrogen peroxide in it, frozen or canned does not.

WATER CARRIES H_2O_2

When they take the water out, yes, God's water in Florida, Texas and California, that little peroxide goes right with it because hydrogen peroxide in the low weak solutions is distillable with water. That's when they don't want to believe me. I've done this test before a scientist from Holland. He said, "I saw it done, but I don't believe it." You can take 1/2% hydrogen peroxide and put it in a retort, boil it, turn it into steam, condense it, and put your potassium iodide in there to liberate enough oxygen to re-ignite the glowing splint. It shouldn't be this way because hydrogen peroxide is supposed to have a boiling point of 152 degrees Fahrenheit. It should be gone like alcohol. It's a quirk in nature. It has to be that way or else life as we know it couldn't be because our body temperature is 98.6. If they say (in error) that hydrogen peroxide boils away at 90 degrees, then there shouldn't be any in our bodies, but there is. Simple, but I guess God meant it that way.

Note: Walter is using the standard potassium iodide test for hydrogen peroxide out of Van Nostrand's Scientific Encyclopedia, 4th. edition. Enough oxygen to re-ignite the splint is not available prior to the adition of the potassium iodide, so it is not ignited by trapped air.

FRUITS AND VEGETABLES

Grapefruit and apple have it. Strawberry doesn't have a whole lot of hydrogen peroxide in it. Watermelon has it. You take the rind and you juice the rind and then run it through, you get a higher percentage yet, because chlorophyll has plenty of oxygen. The photosynthesis process in the green rind liberates it.

Take a raw potato. There is a good amount in it. You take that potato and put it into water and boil it, and then take the water and pour it into the drain. That's when hydrogen peroxide goes with it. It's so soluble, it goes out in the water, and down the drain. Note: This may be why many raw food diets do so well, the peroxide doesn't go down the drain from cooking.

Lettuce doesn't have much hydrogen peroxide in it because the outside leaves are all wilted and you throw them away. There's no chlorophyll left in there. Hydrogen peroxide is in cabbage and tomato, asparagus, green pepper, and watercress.

H_2O_2 DESTROYS HARMFUL MICROORGANISMS

How does this thing work on diseases? When you take it into your body, it raises the oxygen level. Disease germs are mostly anaerobic, which means they cannot live in a high oxygen environment. We told you Dr. Otto Warburg proved that cancer cannot grow in a high oxygen environment. (9) Who is Otto Warburg? He won the Nobel Prize twice. If you get this into your system, it's into your bloodstream. It goes all over your body, it will seek out these microorganisms and destroy them.

Note: Dr. Warburg is sometimes "half" quoted, as saying that: "Oxygen increases the growth rate of cancer cells..." The rest of the sentence is basicly: "just before it kills them."

H_2O_2 TAKES ELECTRONS AWAY FROM GERMS AND VIRUSES, KILLING THEM

Fruton & Simmonds' "General Biochemistry" states that microorganisms themselves possess an electrical charge when suspended in an aqueous medium. Which means when you put them in liquid under a microscope and put two electrical plates in there they will all gravitate to the positive. This tells us they are negatively charged or they contain electrons. Remember the oxygen in hydrogen peroxide is short an electron in it's outer orbit. It will take electrons from whoever donates them. It takes the electrons away from the microorganism. Ask a microbiologist what you have when you take these electrons away, he says you're going to have a dead microorganism. There's a very simple way to prove it.

PROVE TO YOURSELF H_2O_2 KILLS GERMS

Go out and get 1/2 of a test tube of raw fresh milk from the farm. Put in 1/3 teaspoon of 3% hydrogen peroxide. Do the same with either the long shelf life milk or the pasteurized. The milk from the cow will have foam on it in 24 hours. The others won't. We know that raw milk contains microorganisms. That's why we pasteurize. It goes in there, it takes the electrons away from the microorganisms, now it becomes water and oxygen, H_2O and O_2.

This liberated O_2 is not very soluble. It is only soluble 1 part to 32 parts of water at 20 degrees centigrade, or about room temperature. O_2 is not very soluble. It comes up and puts a lot of foam on your milk. Hydrogen peroxide has oxygen in it. The hydrogen peroxide, that one pint bottle you buy in the drug store, is only 3% strength, but has 10 pints of oxygen dissolved in it. When you use the food grade, it's 35% strength, and contains 90 pints (Has 90 pints of oxygen dissolved into it.), and you're only at 35%. That's how soluble it is.

25

ARTHRITIS & CANCER CAUSED BY MICROORGANISMS?

Arthritis caused by a microorganism? On TV there was a doctor standing there saying that arthritis is caused by a virus or a microorganism. This was not news to us.

Arthritis. There is an article out by the Rheumatoid Disease Foundation. (Rte. 4, box 137-OT, Franklin, TN 37064) The article says that we're very suspicious that arthritis is caused by a microorganism. (14)

Note: There is a book available from the Rheumatoid Disease Foundation written by an English doctor, Roger Wyburn-Mason. (14) It details his discovery years ago of an amoeba which causes rheumatoid arthritis. - Sonya C. Starr, B.S., N.C..

Cancer caused by a microorganism? They found out by giving hydrogen peroxide to tiny mice that it doubled their lifespan. (15) The implications for humans is indeed exciting. They put little mice on hydrogen peroxide for two months. They drew blood and the blood oxygen level was higher than they'd ever seen. (21)

Dr. Otto Warburg. What did Dr. Warburg do? He won the Nobel Prize twice. The world recognized what these people did. Dr. Otto Warburg got the Nobel Prize because he proved that cancer cannot grow in a high oxygen environment. (9)

How about cancer? Here's a statement: "Among the most useful carcinogenic agents known at present are several viruses." The author is talking about cancer, he's Dr. James D. Watson. Who's he? He's a famous codiscoverer of the DNA, the double helix. He also won a Nobel Prize with Sir Francis Crick. Crick and Watson. (11)

The book "Cancer - a New Breakthrough." They talk about the cause of cancer. They give electronic microscope pictures of it. They also tell you how contagious it is.

Dr. Eleanor Jackson co-authored the article "A Specific Type of Organism Cultivated From Malignancy: Bacteriology and Proposed Classification." with Virginia Livingston. She gave me her published medical paper on it. (10) She says that the microorganism that causes cancer is so small that it goes through a porcelain filter. They explain how you can isolate it by taking it from a malignant tissue. It's extremely small.

A newspaper article reported that the microorganism that causes Alzheimer's Disease is 100 times smaller than a virus. They thought it was garbage under the electronic microscope until they saw it move. Note: see section on Rife Microscopes.

SIZE OF TINY MICROORGANISMS

How small are viruses? It takes 25,000 human cells stacked up to make one inch. But a virus cannot reproduce, nor can it grow outside of a cell. It will invade a cell, make a nursery out of the cell, and when it explodes, it will release up to 10,000 new viruses. A cubic centimeter will hold 1,000 billion streptococcus microorganisms. That's how small they are.

MUTATING MICROORGANISMS

Microorganisms can change from one disease form into another disease form. Dr. Edward Carl Rosenow did this, and published a paper on it in 1914. He took disease (streptococci or pus) germs, gave them a different food and a different environment and turned up with a different disease (pneumococci or pneumonia) form. Then he reversed the process and came back to the original.

Two microbiologists in New York were reproducing one of the above experiments published by Dr. Rosenow. In her book, "Vaccinations and Injections or Don't Get Stuck", Hannah Allen describes how they took round, berry shaped "cocci" germs, changed their food and changed their environment, and came up with long, rod shaped "bacilli". Then they reversed the process and they changed back to the cocci. These mutations are probably why we're coming up with all these new diseases. Herpes, AIDS, and others. These things can change into something else. Just give them a different environment and different food.
Note: See Rife section.

HOW DO YOU STAY "BUG" FREE?

How can you keep microorganisms out of your body? The first thing to do is to keep your body healthy. That is by a proper diet. If somebody told me two years ago that hydrogen peroxide and diet were interconnected, I would have told them no way. But they are. Note: See section on Macrobiotics.

COLON

Also, a good cleansing program to get your body cleaned up is good. Look into the V. E. Irons program. He spoke in Pittsburgh, where I saw him. He checked in right after me. He didn't even have a wrinkle in his face, he's 89 years old. He's got a son that is 64. Whatever he's doing, he's doing it right.

Note: The reader may want to investigate the book "Tissue Cleansing Through Bowel Management" by Dr. Bernard Jensen. - Available from: Colema Boards, Inc. P.O. Box 229-OT, Anderson, CA 96007. Also please refer to the section in this book: "A Clean Bowel".

ANIMALS

Do any of your pets have arthritis or tumors?. I know of a cow that's got leukemia. It didn't eat for two weeks. It was given hydrogen peroxide and is eating hay and grain again.

HOUSEPLANTS

Try hydrogen peroxide on your houseplants. Take 1 ounce to a quart of water and water your houseplants with it. Watch what they do.

My neighbor and good friend, in March of last year, tore branches off of a lilac bush, put them in a bucket, supported them, and put a solution of hydrogen peroxide in it. The bush bloomed purple blossoms for Easter.

The point is, that plants need hydrogen peroxide. If you go to a spring and find watercress growing, you can rest assured that spring has a high hydrogen peroxide content. Watercress does not root in the ground, it roots in the water. All roots have to have oxygen. Watercress gets the oxygen out of the water.

GETTING HARDER TO CURE ILLNESSES

Dr. Max Gerson said that 25 years hence there is going to be more cancer and it's going to be harder to cure. He said this is because our air is not what it used to be. Our water is not what it used to be, and our food is not what it used to be.

MICROORGANISMS ON OUR FOOD ARE HARDY

There are microorganisms in your food. If you think that just because you cooked your food you killed the microorganisms, this is not so. Some microorganisms can withstand temperatures down to 190 degrees below 0. Some can take temperatures up to 126 degrees above. Water boils at 100 degrees centigrade. In order to kill them, they have to autoclave them in boiling water for 96 hours. That's how tough they are. They have found them in the deepest sediment of the ocean. They have found them on the highest mountain. They are all over. They have been around a long time, But they can't stand a high amount of oxygen.

WARTS

Warts and moles are caused by a virus. I found a medical paper. The title of it is "The Simple and Painless Treatment of Warts." It said to gently cut them open & put a drop of H_2O_2 inside, killing the virus.

HOW OFTEN DO YOU TAKE H_2O_2?

Question: Do you take it everyday? Answer: I didn't take it after I went through the program for six months to see whether or not my arthritis would come back. It didn't. I took it every time I felt a cold or flu coming on. The next morning I had no problem.

AVAILABILITY

Question: Where do you get reagent grade hydrogen peroxide? Answer: The druggist. He can get it for you if he wants to. He can call a supplier. It is what is used by medical people. The food grade is much cheaper, about $12 a pint.

PERMEATES POLYETHELENE

In the Aseptic Packaging Process, the inner liner of the juice carton is polyethelene, the second layer is aluminum, then two layers of cardboard, and a finish on the outside. Oxygen permeates polyethelene. You can take a polyethelene bottle, put in 35%

hydrogen peroxide, and leave it in the refrigerator for a month. Come back and put your hands on it. They'll turn white. The oxygen is clinging to the outside of the bottle. In the aseptic package, they spray the inside of the box with H_2O_2 and if it wasn't for the foil, it would keep right on going out.

PRESERVING

Question: What are the ramifications of using it for home preserving? Answer: Some people are trying it. There are some tests going on now. They are taking strawberries and blueberries and things like that. You rinse them off with hydrogen peroxide and cap them up in a jar and keep them refrigerated. They also tried sweetcorn the same way. There are a lot of experimental things being done.

METHODS OF USING H_2O_2

You can get hydrogen peroxide into your body in a number of ways. If you've got foot problems, you could soak your feet in a warmed 3% solution. When you shower, you can spray your body with the 3%. Be careful to keep away from around your eyes. You could brush your teeth with 3%.

PLAQUE FROM MICROORGANISMS

Question: What causes plaque? A microorganism. Deposits, just like coral in the sea, are made by a microorganism. We've got medical articles here telling about how H_2O_2 will dissolve plaque. (6) I chipped plaque away from my teeth, dropped it in a test tube, put some 3% in and it boiled and disappeared.

H_2O_2 MANUFACTURE

Question: What is peroxide made from? Answer: Commercially, they take barium peroxide and treat it with sulfuric acid. Then they distill the peroxide away. There are other ways to make it. You can make it with ozone. You can make it with electricity. Charging plates underwater will turn the water into hydrogen peroxide, but the percentage will not get very high. By using the plates, I think they can get up to about 20%. All they are doing is just adding that extra oxygen on. $2H_2O \rightarrow H_2O_2 + H_2\char`\^$

GROTZ DIETARY PREFERENCES

I'm more careful of what I eat. I like salads, I eat a lot of fresh fruit. I stay away from sugar. Blackstrap molasses? It's quite natural. It has not been interfered with by man too much. Eat foods that are the least interfered with by man. A good example is eating butter over margarine. Margarine has been hydrogenated. They pass hydrogen through the oils to make it solid. The body has never been able to digest it properly.

U.S.A. HEALTH DECLINES

41 million Americans have serious arthritis. 20 million have herpes. 13 million have diabetes. That's 74 million people, over a third of our population, and I've only covered three diseases. At the beginning of this century we had the healthiest nation on earth. We're now the wealthiest, but far from the healthiest.

HIGH BLOOD PRESSURE

High blood pressure. A man had a triple bypass, and couldn't leave his house because his blood pressure was so high. He heard about this hydrogen peroxide. He went to his doctor and had a physical examination, and says he's going to have his blood pressure monitored every other day. He did so. His blood pressure went down to where it was when he was in high school. He's back on the road giving lectures again.

DOCTOR APOLOGIZES TO CANCER PATIENT

Cancer. I have a neighbor who started taking hydrogen peroxide about a month after I did. She was given two months to live by the Mayo Clinic. She should have been dead in June of 1982. She went back to Mayo and told them she was on peroxide, and the doctor was furious. Her daughter was there and said, "Look, doctor, this is my mother you're talking to." She said, "I have this booklet I want you to read." She gave her doctor some of Dr. Rosenow's papers. The doctor said " Oh, he's a colleague of mine." He came back later and apologized. He said, "Go on taking it, it's not going to hurt you." But, he said, "If you get well you're not going to know if it's the peroxide that did it or the radiation." Her daughter replied "That's all right, doctor, you won't know either if it's the radiation or the peroxide".

H_2O_2 VITALIZES OVERWORKED IMMUNE SYSTEM

In my opinion, hydrogen peroxide is part of the immune system of the body. Our bodies don't make enough hydrogen peroxide to counteract the polluted air or water or germs we take in. We have to counteract what we take in. While the body is busy taking care of that, guess who's setting up housekeeping? All the pathogenic microorganisms.

PEOPLE DRANK H_2O_2 IN 1926

I got a call from California from a man who was very close to Dr. Virginia Livingston. He said: "Do you people think you've got something new?" I said: No. I know I don't. It's very old. He said: "That's right. I have a book I'm going to send you from 1926 that talks about the drinking of hydrogen peroxide. Dr. William Frederick Koch from Detroit, Michigan, who taught medicine at Wayne State University. Back in the early 30's he was curing cancer."

COMPUTER SEARCH FINDS HISTORICAL RESEARCH

Computer search... We put in hydrogen peroxide and human blood. 33 articles came out. Last September a lady from South Dakota called me and asked: "Do you have any medical articles on hydrogen peroxide and leukemia?" I said No. She asked if I could get some for her. I told her I'd share the expense of a computer search. 26 articles came out. When I put my order in, the girl said: Hey, what's going on with this hydrogen peroxide business? She said: You're the third person today that has put an order in for a computer search on hydrogen peroxide, and one of them was a law firm. A law firm? It must be interesting.

In October we put in just, "hydrogen peroxide", that's all, to see how much material is in there. In the last 19 years there were 3,690 published medical articles. A doctor told me that of all the material submitted, less than 15% becomes published. The medical computer only goes back to 1966. The oldest medical article we have is September 1884. You are looking at a period of about 80 years that you have to do by hand. There are some terrific ones in there. Like out of the Lancet, how in 1919 they were injecting it into people during the big flu epidemic. The Lancet is the British equivalent of our AMA Journal. It tells in the article how over 80% of the people were dying in one ward where they had the influenza cases. (13)

I thought I better look at ozone, too, because they are closely related. I went into the computer again to see what was there. In the last 19 years there were 895 published medical articles on it. Without exaggeration I will be able to produce a listing naming over 5,000 articles done on it, when I combine hydrogen peroxide and ozone in a search of the last 100 years. What are we going to do? Are we going to wait until another 5,000 articles are published? Think of the money this costs.

Ozone. Dr. Puharich holds the patent on the treatment of cancerous tumors with ozone. He injects right into the tumor. He gave a seminar. I was asked by the sponsors to come and give a brief comment. Dr. Puharich insisted I speak first. Ozone. It has the same problem as hydrogen peroxide. The material cost to treat a cancerous tumor with ozone is four cents.

Ozone is going to rapidly be replacing our chlorine. Ozone in water can kill bacteria 5,000 times faster than chlorine. It also kills waterborne viruses and waterborne parasites. Chlorine can react with organic matter in our drinking water to form carcinogens. Los Angeles is going to spend 120 million dollars to ozonate their water. In my own state of Minnesota, there's a city that has already got their ozonator waiting to be put into operation. Potsdam, New York and Casper, Wyoming have ozonators as well. A total of 18 cities in the U.S. now use ozone, and Europe has 3,000. Note: See sections on Medical and Industrial Ozone.

MULTIPLE SCLEROSIS

I am surprised that people with multiple sclerosis have never been told of the hyperbaric oxygen chamber. It is in the New England Journal of Medicine. (18)

GERMAN LAW REQUIRES DOCTORS INFORM YOU OF NUTRITION ALTERNATIVES

I love the law that's on the national books in West Germany. If you have cancer your doctor must, under the law of West Germany, tell you your four alternatives. Surgery, chemotherapy, radiation, and <u>nutrition</u>.

- End of Walter Grotz's talk.

E.C.H.O. SUPPLIED REFERENCES
(Proof Supplied For W. Grotz's Claims In Previous Section)

1. Subject: **"Penicillium"** (Penicillium Notatin) (Gen Biochemistry, Fruton & Simmonds 577.1 F 944 p. 339) "Since the oxidation of glucose by O2 in the presence of penicillium notatin results in the formation of bactericidal amounts of H_2O_2."

2. Subject: **"Interferon"** (IFN) (Journal of Interferon Research Vol. 3 Number 2 1983 p. 143-151) "The results suggest then that IFN may stimulate the production of low amounts of H_2O_2 and possibly other oxygen intermediates (OH) which are a necessary event early in the pathway of IFN activation of human NK cells." (NK-Natural Killer) "We present evidence here which is compatible with the suggestion that H_2O_2 and possible other oxygen intermediates, may also play a role in the IFN-mediated augmentation of cytolytic function in another effector cell type, the human killer (NK) cell." "These results raise the possibility that the chemiluminesence response generated by IFN may be due to the liberation of H_2O_2, OH, and possible other oxygen intermediates."

3. Subject: **"Hydrogen Peroxide Mediated Killing of Bacteria"** (Molecular & Cellular Biochemistery 49, 143-149 (1982) "Polymorphonuclear leukcytes (PMN) or neutrophils have multiple systems available for killing ingested bacteria. Nearly each of these incorporates H_2O_2 indicating the essential nature of this reactive oxygen intermediate for microbicidal activity." "These mechanisms appear important since deficiencies of H_2O_2 production, myeloperoxidase or lactoferrin frequently increases their owner's susceptibility to infection."

4. Subject: **"Hydrogen Peroxide Release from Human Blood Platelets"** Allesandro Finazzi-Agro, Institute of Biochemistry, University of Rome, Biochimica et Biophysica Acta, 718 (1982) p.21-25. "In this paper we report on H_2O_2 release by platelets when challenged by particulate membrane-perturbing agents."

5.   Subject: **"Cell Division in Normal and Transformed Cells: the Possible role of Superoxide and Hydrogen Peroxide"**. Oberley, Oberley, and Buettner. Medical Hypotheses 7: p.21-42 (1981) "We hypothesize that H_2O_2 is the ultimate cause of normal cell division."

6.   Subject: **"Removal of Cholesterol and Other Lipids from Experimental Animal and Human Atheromatous Arteries by Dilute Hydrogen Peroxide"**. "In vitro studies conducted with human aorta incubated with dilute hydrogen peroxide for various periods of time demonstrated the elution (extracting by means of a solvent) cholesterol, esters, phospholipids, triglycerides, and free fatty acids from the arterial wall." (Baylor University Medical Center, Dallas Texas.) Authors: James W. Finney, M.A., Bruce E. Jay, B.S., George J. Race, M.D., Harold C. Urschel, M.D., John T. Mallams, M.D. and George A. Balla, M.D., F.I.C.A., U.S.P.H.S. Grants.

7.   Subject: **"Generation of H_2O_2 in Biomembranes"**. T. Ramasarma: Biochimica et Biophysica Acta 694 (1982) p.69-93 Elsevier Biomedical Press; Department of Biochemistry, Indian Institute of Science, Bangalore 560 012. "Thus, the generation of H_2O_2 in cellular processes seems to be purposeful and H_2O_2 cannot be dismissed as a mere undesirable byproduct... The capacity for generation of H_2O_2 is now found to be widespread in a variety of organisms and in the organelles of the cells."

8.   Subject: **"Killing of Blood-Stage Murine Malaria Parasites by Hydrogen Peroxide"**. (Infection and Immunity. Jan. 1983 p.456-459). "A Radical Interpretation of Immunity to Malaria Parasites" (The Lancet Dec. 25, 1982 p.1431-1433) "Free Oxygen Radical Generators as Antimalorial Drugs" (The Lancet Jan. 29, 1983 p.359-360)

9.   Subject: **"The Prime Cause and Prevention of Cancer With Two Prefaces on Prevention"**. Author: Dr. Otto Warburg; twice Nobel Laureate. Malignant cancer cells are anaerobic (live without oxygen) and cannot live in a high oxygen environment.

10.   Subject: **"A Specific Type of Organism Cultivated from Malignancy: Bacteriology and Proposed Classification"**. Authors: Virginia Wuerthele-Casoe Livingston, M.D. & Eleanor Alexander-Jackson, Ph.D.

11.   Subject: **"Molecular Biology of the Gene"**. Author: Dr. James D. Watson, Nobel Laureate, Codiscoverer of the DNA double Helix. A geneticist's view of cancer page 469. "Among the most useful carcinogenic agents known at present are several viruses."

12.   Subject: **"Diseases of Birds"**. "Stroud's Digest on the Diseases of Birds" Author: Robert Stroud; "The Birdman of Alcatraz" What did the "Birdman of Alcatraz" Robert Stroud use to cure the birds? - Sodium perborate and hydrogen peroxide and sodium perborate in water gives you hydrogen peroxide.

13.   Subject: **Influenzal Pneumonia: The Intravenous Injection of Hydrogen Peroxide.** Speaking of an epidemic of pneumonia cases: "The mortality (48%) compares very favorably with the 80% in similar cases not so treated, and more so when it is remembered

that we only treated the most severe and apparently hopeless."
Also: 1. Hydrogen peroxide can be given intravenously without gas
embolism being produced. 2. The anoxaemia is often markedly
benefited. 3. The toxaemia appears to be overcome in many cases.
The Lancet, Feb 21, 1920. Drs. T. H. Oliver & D. V. Murphy.

14. Subject: **"Oxygen"** - O_2 **The Life-Giving Element**, Roger
Wyburn-Mason (an English Doctor) discovered an amoeba which causes
rheumatoid arthritis. The Nutrition and Dietary Consultant, Sonya
C. Starr, B.S., N.C.

15. Subject: **"Cumulative Data & Experimental Results of first 8
Experiments 3/25-8/30 1982"** Mice with "growth to a much larger size
and an almost doubled lifespan" due to H_2O_2. Winifred Wirth, Iowa
Conference on Hydrogen Peroxide, Sept. 12, 1983. Her studies
started at St. Thomas Institute, Cincinnati OH, and concluded at
Columbia University, 1980, Dr. Winifred Wirth, Ph.D. in
Bacteriology. Final results published by the Cardiff (in-Wales)
Medical School. Distributed by the Catholic Health Organization.

16. Subject: **"The Effects of Hydrogen Peroxide on the Ehrlich
Carcinoma in Laboratory Mice: St. Thomas Institute, Cincinnati,
Ohio; Nov 15, 1982"**. "The oral administration of hydrogen
peroxide... was effective in the treatment of mice bearing the
Ehrlich carcinoma as judged by mortality and delay in palpable
tumor incidence."

17. Subject: **"Oxygen for Prevention of Wound Infection"** Knighton,
et al. Arch Surg. 119:199-204, 1984 "Oxygen therapy appears to be
as effective as antibiotic prophylaxis."

18. Subject: **"Hyperbaric-Oxygen treatment of Multiple Sclerosis"**
Boguslav H Fischer, M.D., Morton Marks, M.D., and Theobald Reich,
M. D. The New England Journal of Medicine, January 27, 1983, Vol.
308, No. 4.

19. Subject: **"Vitamin U Concentrate Therapy of Peptic Ulcer"**
Garnett Cheney, M.D. The American Journal of Gastroenterology,
March, 1954.

20. Subject: **"Leukocyte-Generated Hydrogen Peroxide Depression of
Cardiac Sarcoplasmic Reticulum Calcium Transport - A Hypothetical
Effector Mechanism of Rejection"** " It is hypothesized that oxygen
free radicals and hydrogen peroxide may play a major role in...
cardiac rejection..." Transplantation 1983 July; 36 (1) p. 117-119.

21. Subject: **"The Supersaturation of Biologic Fluids With Oxygen
by the Decomposition of Hydrogen Peroxide"** "Preliminary data were
obtained from blood, plasma or other catalase-containing fluids
from experimental animals and human beings. The findings suggest
that these fluids become "supersaturated" with oxygen following
their breakdown of exogenous hydrogen peroxide." Jay, Finney,
Balla, & Mallams (Baylor University) Texas Report Biol. & Med.,
22:106.1964

Walter Grotz just spent 2 1/2 months writing eighteen hours a day, compiling H_2O_2 information for the U.S. Congress - Office of Technology Assessment. In July 1988 he sent a 50 pound package of hydrogen peroxide information to them to be assessed. The assessors are composed of 19 members, 1/2 orthodox, 1/2 alternative. He did this only to help the good of the whole. He was neither required to, or paid to, he was requested to. They are supposed to assess it by December, 1988. Walter hopes they read the whole 50 pounds.

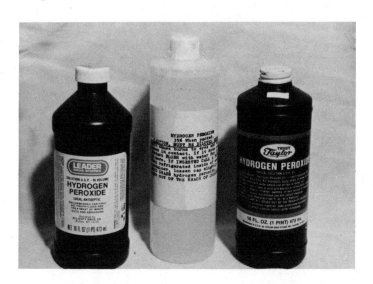

3% DRUGSTORE PEROXIDE VS. 35% FOOD GRADE

GRADES OF H2O2

3%   **Drug/Grocery.** Also contains "stabilizers" like: phenol, acetanilide, acetanilid, sodium stanate, tetrasodium phosphate.

6%   **Beautician** Grade. Stabilizers unknown.

30%   **Reagent** hydrogen peroxide. Medical research grade, contains stabilizers.

30-32% Electronic Grade. Stabilizers unknown.

35%   **Technical** Grade, contains small amount of phosphorous to neutralize chlorine.

35%   **Food** Grade, also 50% Food Grade. Used in food.

90%   **Rocket fuel.**

99.6% **Pure Experimental** Grade.

ADDITIONAL USES FOR 35% FOOD GRADE HYDROGEN PEROXIDE

Caution: If you spill 35% H_2O_2 on your skin, rinse immediately with water. Avoid any contact with eyes.

*To make a 3% solution: mix 1 oz. 35% to 11 ozs. water. Use distilled water as often as possible.

Vegetable soak: Add ½ cup 3% H_2O_2 to a full sink of cold water. Soak light skinned (like lettuce) 20 minutes, thicker skinned (like cucumbers) 30 minutes. Drain, dry and refrigerate. Prolongs freshness.

If time is a problem, spray vegetables (and fruits) with a solution of 3%. Let stand for a few minutes, rinse and dry.

Leftover tossed salad: Spray with a solution of ½ cup water and 1 Tbsp. 3%. Drain, cover and refrigerate.

To freshen kitchen: Keep a spray bottle of 3% in the kitchen. Use it to wipe off counter tops and appliances. It will disinfect and give the kitchen a fresh smell. Works great in the refrigerator and kid's school lunch boxes.

Marinade: Place meat, fish, or poultry in a casserole (avoid using aluminum pans). Cover with 3% H_2O_2. Place loosely covered in refrigerator for ½ hour. Rinse and cook.

In the dishwasher: Add 2 ozs. of 3% H_2O_2 to your regular washing formula.

Sprouting seeds: Add 1 oz. 3% H_2O_2 to 1 pint of water and soak the seeds overnight. Add the same amount of H_2O_2 each time you rinse the seeds.

House and garden plants: Put 1 oz. 3% H_2O_2 in 1 quart water. (Or add 16 drops 35% to one quart water.) Water or mist plants with this solution.

Insecticide spray: Mix 8 ozs. white sugar, 4-8 ozs. 3% H_2O_2 in 1 gallon of water.

Humidifiers and steamers: Mix 1 pint 3% H_2O_2 to 1 gallon of water.

Laundry: Add 8 ozs. of 3% to your wash in place of bleaches.

Shower: Keep a spray bottle of 3% H_2O_2 in the shower. Spray your body after washing to replace the acid mantle on your skin that soap removes.

Facial: Use 3% on a cotton ball as a facial freshener after washing.

Rejuvenating Detoxifying bath: Add 6 ozs. 35% H_2O_2 to ½ tub of water. May increase H_2O_2 up to 2 cups per bath. Soak at least ½ hour.

Alternate bath: Add ½ cup 35% H_2O_2, ½ cup sea salt, ½ cup baking soda or epsom salts to bath water and soak.

Foot soak: Add 1½ ozs. 35% H_2O_2 to 1 gallon water and soak.

Athlete's foot: Soak feet nightly in 3% H_2O_2 until condition is improved.

Mouthwash: Use 3% H_2O_2. Add a dash of liquid chlorophyll for flavoring if desired.

Toothpaste: Use baking soda and add enough 3% H_2O_2 to make a paste. Or just dip your brush in 3% H_2O_2 and brush.

Douche or Enema: Add 6 Tbls. of 3% H_2O_2 to a quart of distilled water. 6 Tbls. is *the maximum amount to use.*

Colonic: Add ½ pint 3% H_2O_2 to 5 gallons warm water. (Note: 1 pint 3% is *the maximum amount to use.*)

Pets: For small animals (dogs & cats) use 1 oz. 3% H_2O_2 to 1 qt. of water.

Agriculture: Use 8 ozs. 35% H_2O_2 per 1000 gallons of water. If you do not have an injector, start out by using 1 tsp. 35% H_2O_2 in the drinking cup at the stanchion.

For the drinking water of cows that are sick, use 1 pt. 3% H_2O_2 to 5 gallons of water. To drench sick calves, put 1/3 pt. of 3% H_2O_2 in a pt. bottle and fill remainder with water. Do this twice a day. For an adult cow, use the same procedure, but use a quart.

To foliage feed crops, put 5 to 16 ozs. of 35% food grade hydrogen peroxide into 20 gallons of water. Spray on plants early in the morning when the dew is still on them and the birds are singing. (It has been found that the singing of the birds opens the pores of the plants.)

36

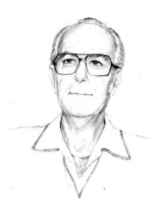

DR. CHARLES H. FARR, M.S., Ph.D., M.D.

Our next speaker will be Dr. Farr. But first, a discussion. Dr. Farr studied at the Oklahoma School of Medicine, and has practiced since 1962. He is the founder of the International Academy of Bio-Oxidative Medicine. He is a member of the A.M.A., the American Association for Advancement of Science, Oklahoma Academy of Science, Sigma XI, Southwestern Section Society of Experimental Biology and Medicine, New York Academy of Sciences, American College for Advancement in Medicine, International Academy of Preventive Medicine, Academy of Metabiology and the American Holistic Medical Association. He has authored over 31 scientific and medical publications, and has been awarded many honors.

Dr. Farr takes a different viewpoint than both our previous speakers, advocating caution in taking hydrogen peroxide by mouth, and preferring only the intravenous methods. He has published a paper entitled "Oral Hydrogen Peroxide - Killer Or Cure??". In it, he states:

"Our body has a very poor tolerance to hydrogen peroxide when taken orally... The levels of the enzymes, Catalase and Glutathione Peroxidase are so tiny in gastric (stomach) juice, that only very small amounts of hydrogen peroxide, when taken orally, would be converted into water and oxygen... There is a growing legion of people who are anxious to testify to the alleged healing power of hydrogen peroxide when taken by mouth. The freedom which allows them to express their convictions, allows you to collect adequate knowledge and make an intelligent decision about your own health care... Hydrogen peroxide is proving beneficial when given intravenously by a trained physician."

Dr. Farr states we don't know enough, yet, about the purely biochemical, long term results of drinking dilute solutions of hydrogen peroxide to trust it. Still, on the other side of this "what if?" equation, are the many people with "terminal" illnesses who have used it with benefit, and as of yet, show no side effects. Add to that, the body of knowledge starting to emerge from publications in the 20's & 30's showing no harm, and we have quite a lot of weight on the side of oral usage.

37

This particular controversy seems to be brewing between oral peroxide actual users and people who aren't. The proponents have used hydrogen peroxide orally for years, and generally swear that it removed, or reduced, all sorts of afflictions, without causing any harm. These are usually honest, respectable, average people, who were in a tight spot, and found relief in oral hydrogen peroxide use after other methods had failed. In fairness, we must consider that there exists the possibility of a small percentage of this group being over zealous and non professional. On the other side, we have the non-users. The non-users say we should look at scientific theory and various "test tube" studies, and conclude that oral ingestion must be dangerous. Most of the "anti" oral usage group appear to be honest, respectable, well meaning and prudent people, who, for safety reasons, would prefer to err on the side of caution, if at all. Still, on this side of the argument too, we must be cautious, because in any group there is usually a small percentage who's motives might solely be to protect their own financial interests from competition. I am not referring to Dr. Farr, a cautious man. Evaluate all, and make up your own mind.

The very existence of this controversy is proof that we have to move away from theory on both sides, and into large, controlled, and unbiased clinical trials of every major oxygenation method mentioned in this book. We also have to follow up on all the people we can find who already experienced these methods. Perhaps it will end up being discovered that there are, as yet, undiscovered factors at work in our amazingly adaptive bodies, that allow us to occasionally drink dilute solutions of food grade hydrogen peroxide without harm. Now, on to Dr. Farr's talk.

EXCERPTS FROM TALK BY DR. CHARLES H. FARR:
INTRAVENOUS AND OTHER USES OF HYDROGEN PEROXIDE

Please be seated. We're going to talk about a very interesting substance. It's called hydrogen peroxide. Hydrogen peroxide in early times was used as rocket fuel, as you may be aware.

Let me give a little background. I'm both MD and Ph.D. Ph.D. in biochemistry, MD in practicing medicine. My interest has always been in trying to do something, or find out what I can do, to preserve life. Because we know that disease is the opposite of health. When you're not healthy, you're diseased. If we can possibly reestablish your health, you're going to have less disease. One thing has always caught the interest of physicians who work with chronic degenerative diseases, oxygen.

Oxygen is needed in the body. We can be without food and water for a lengthy time. We can be without oxygen only for a few seconds. I think of it as the spark of life.

We're going to play scientist. Every one of you in this room, obviously, is a researcher like myself. I say that because if you weren't you wouldn't be in this room. You're curious. You want to learn something about what is happening to your environment and what you can do. That is basically what research is. It is curiosity. Wanting to learn. Then trying to find out.

We're going to talk about oxygen. If we're going to do some real basic research, we have to go down to the very lowest form. The molecular form. The atom form would have a nucleus and some electrons spinning around it. If we look at this atom in another way, we might see that at the top we have a hydrogen atom, which is a very small atom. Now let's look at something called an oxygen atom.

FREE RADICAL OXYGEN

In this case, singlet oxygen. It means there is just one unit. That one unit may be toxic to you by itself. I'm sure you've all heard of free radical oxygen. Free radical oxygen is a singlet oxygen with one electron removed. Below that we have an oxygen molecule. This is the stuff that we know is good for us. We think that it is. A lot of doctors look at oxygen as a toxic substance, because of what happens to it. It breaks down into these free radicals.

If we take the singlet oxygen of the second atom, add two atoms of hydrogen to it, we have water, $H_2 + O$. Water is a, chemically, very well balanced molecule. It is stable. It doesn't break down. It doesn't tear itself up.

Now we have ozone. I'm sure some of you have heard about ozone. It has been used therapeutically for many years. You'll notice through that diagram of a molecule, there are two red lines which show the lines of cleavage. One molecule is very, very unstable. In fact, the ozone molecule reacts with hydrogen to form hydrogen peroxide. When physicians are treating you with ozone, the end effect of that probably is hydrogen peroxide, thereby giving you this therapeutic value. Note: there is discussion over this, going on too. Many compounds are formed, and science is trying to sort it out.

The last molecule is hydrogen peroxide. You'll see there are also two lines of cleavage to that molecule. Two atoms of oxygen and two atoms of hydrogen, H_2O_2. It's made up from one molecule of water and one additional singlet oxygen atom, $H_2O + O$. It's also a very unstable molecule, it breaks down slowly, by itself, through a process called dismutation. It just means it falls apart. In the body, hydrogen peroxide falls apart and produces water and oxygen. $H_2O_2 > H_2O + O$. We say, that's great. That's what we need. We need some of this oxygen. In the body it requires an enzyme.

CATALASE

In fact, there are a number of enzymes that are involved with hydrogen peroxide, but the most important one, the most common one, is called catalase. The purpose of the catalase in the body is to take the hydrogen peroxide and break it down into water and oxygen.

We just took some hydrogen peroxide liquid; very weak, dilute
solution, and we put a drop or two of blood in it. After about one
minute we don't see much happening. Some very tiny bubbles come up
there. They're coming off because the catalase enzyme in the blood
is converting the hydrogen peroxide into oxygen and water. At
three minutes I think it's very obvious to you. It is breaking it
down. At five minutes even more so. It looks like it's boiling.
Ten minutes later, the activity is virtually gone. The waste is in
the bottom. The blood is still there. It didn't go anywhere. It
didn't dissolve. It was the catalase in the blood that converted
the hydrogen peroxide into oxygen and water. It quit after about
two minutes because we used up all the catalase enzyme. That's
important in the test tube, but how important is it in your body?

PEROXISOMES - HUMAN CELLS PRODUCE H_2O_2

Every cell contains small bodies within the cell. Those
bodies have various names, depending on what they do. Some are
called the nuclei, some are lysosomes, some mitochondria, they have
all kinds of different names. In there, one is called a
peroxisome.

The specific purpose of this peroxisome in the cells of your
body is to produce hydrogen peroxide. Why? What is its purpose?
It is amazing as you read through the literature about hydrogen
peroxide, you'll find it being called the left-over product or the
by-product or the waste-product of metabolism. We're going to have
to completely change your mind about this marvelous molecule.

WHITE CELLS

The first line of defense in the body is your white cells.
Your white cells, the little soldiers as they're talked about,
engulf things in your body that shouldn't be there. Those may be
bacteria, protozoa, or yeast. The complexes, the things that cause
you to have allergy reactions, the viruses. I don't feel that
hydrogen peroxide directly in any way destroys a virus, but it
inhibits its action. That is another mechanism, we'll talk about
it another time. White cells close around a particle, whatever
that particle is. Peroxisomes first come out of the white cells,
and then, they go into a compartment in the white cell, right along
with the particles that the white cells have eaten. All of a
sudden, the engulfed peroxisomes and particles disappear. Why they
disappear, is because the peroxisome produced hydrogen peroxide in
there to destroy that particle, whether that's a bacteria, or
whatever is foreign to your body. This is your very first line of
defense. Your own body produces hydrogen peroxide as part of the
immune system.

Let's say there are 10,000 of those bacterial particles out
there around one white cell. What do you think its capacity may
be? It certainly can't eat 10,000. If we think about hydrogen
peroxide as being produced by the white cells, it is the first line
of defense to destroy these substances. Under certain conditions,
you can have many, many more of these foreign substances, such as
bacteria, in your body than your white cells can take care of.

40

This is where we start getting into some rationale to say, "what if we use hydrogen peroxide in larger amounts, put it in the vein to kill off the excess bacteria?" That's where this starts coming from. What if?

FIRST INTRAVENOUS USE 1920

(Note: W. Grotz mentioned this, too.) The very first article I found in the literature that directly relates to the intravenous use of hydrogen peroxide is this one. Published in the Lancet in 1920 by Dr. Oliver. What was happening was that they were having a very severe influenza pneumonia type of problem. In this particular area in India, the death rate was around 80%. He reasoned that these people had pneumonia. They could not get enough oxygen, so maybe by giving them hydrogen peroxide he would be giving them some oxygen. Sounds logical doesn't it? He concocted a setup to produce hydrogen peroxide chemically. He infused these people and the death rate dropped 48%. Half. It is amazing that something that startling could have been done in 1920 and totally ignored all these years and never looked at again. What do you think happened? These people had bacterial infections, viral infections. There were a mixed bunch of infections in the body giving them this very severe high death rate, influenza - pneumonia type problem. The hydrogen peroxide must have done something.

Dr. Oliver stated, and I totally agree with him, that there was not enough oxygen produced in the hydrogen peroxide to do any good, really. He said it must be that the hydrogen peroxide oxidized, or burned back, the part with toxins. Burned up the bacteria. Killed the bacteria. It was an extremely astute observation.

RESEARCH IN THE 50'S & 60'S

Through the 50's and 60's there were a lot of doctors who became interested in hydrogen peroxide, because they felt the same way. If we give hydrogen peroxide, we will produce oxygen. Oxygen is known to sensitize, as an example, cancer tissue. Because most of the cancer cells live in an anaerobic or, "without oxygen" state. If you give them a big dose of oxygen, you may help do something. The big interest was in using x-ray to try to kill cancer and they found that if they could give some hydrogen peroxide along with the x-ray, the killing effect of the x-ray was magnified. It was a little better. There was a lot of interest there.

They were using this intra-arterially. You have an artery every place in your body. You have one that goes out to each arm, one to each leg. They were shooting it into the artery to go out to the cancer. If you have cancer out in your fingers, they would shoot it into the arm to go out to that cancer. They were using it only intra-arterially. They measured the amount of oxygen being produced.

HYPERBARIC OXYGEN

Are any of you familiar with hyperbaric oxygen, also called HBO, where we used a tank? Those tanks cost anywhere from $70,000 to $106,000. I used to have a couple of them. They are explosive. They are dangerous in many ways. They can burst your eardrums and so forth. But still, there is a lot of benefit that comes from hyperbaric oxygen.

One of the doctors measured the amount of oxygen produced in tissue within hyperbaric chambers. He found the limit was 200 units. He gave intravenous hydrogen peroxide and measured how much it produced. It produced 300. They have a $70,000 expensive, potentially dangerous tank, producing 200 units of oxygen. Over here you have $.03 worth of hydrogen peroxide producing one third more. NOTE: See section on HBO.

EARLY EXPERIMENTS TOO SHORT

I keep exploring the literature on hydrogen peroxide. I ran across this article. An article done by Gymon, middle 60's. They likewise, were measuring the oxygen content produced by hydrogen peroxide. They had measured the tissue. What they were doing was giving the hydrogen peroxide in the artery. They would put a probe in there to measure how much oxygen was being produced. They found that some very interesting things happened. They said that if we measure three different people, we get three different patterns. There is no consistency to it. Here is the arterial amount, and here is the tissue amount. They correspond pretty well sometimes. Other times they don't. Other times they don't at all. Their conclusion was, don't fool around with hydrogen peroxide, just give them some oxygen with the mask. That's all you have to do, just give them oxygen. That got me thinking, because those experiments only went on for about 35-40 minutes.

Other articles were published that said: We found that there is a substance in the body called cytochrome C which you have heard about. This cytochrome C mixes with hydrogen peroxide and forms a stable complex. That complex is there for at least 40 minutes or longer, before it starts breaking down. After about 30 minutes the cytochrome C starts acting like catalase. Remember, catalase breaks down hydrogen peroxide. What's happening here is, obviously, after 35 or 40 minutes, you're getting some boiling action from catalase, as well as cytochrome C breaking down the hydrogen peroxide. It's not a simple thing at all. You don't simply take hydrogen peroxide and split it up into oxygen and water. It's very complicated. In the red cell alone, the oxygen and peroxide get involved in all kinds of metabolism. Peroxide has to be active in there. It's not just a simple reaction. We studied it some more and found that they said, Well, we'll do it intra-arterially, since it dissolves cholesterol and triglycerides, and is good for arteriosclerotic diseases. It has certain demonstrative effects on the white cells and the platelets.

The old ideas were that hydrogen peroxide was simple. It broke down very easily, into water and oxygen. If you put it in the body, it breaks down very quickly.

In fact, most studies showed that it might break down in as little as two seconds or less. When broken down, you have nothing but oxygen. No hydrogen peroxide left.

We actually found, with cytochrome C, the injected hydrogen peroxide lasted up to 40 minutes. It came back to the heart and the lungs. What happens to it there? It "boiled" off. You have oxygen in your blood. Excess oxygen comes around to the lungs. It comes off. I know all you scientists know what the lungs look like. To get into the lungs, it comes in through the pulmonary artery into the alveoli, the little air sacs. Everyone assumes the oxygen comes out there, that it doesn't go any farther. That's what everyone is thinking. We said: Something's wrong.

First of all, there is evidence that it lasts 30 minutes not just 12 seconds or 2 seconds. Secondly, if that oxygen was coming off of the lungs, there should be some way to measure that. What do you do when you measure oxygen consumption? You measure metabolic rate. By measuring the amount of oxygen breathed in, and subtracting from it the amount breathed out, we can measure metabolic rate. You would think that if the hydrogen peroxide's oxygen was coming out into the lungs, it would be exhaled, and we'd have a negative amount in our equation, more coming out than going in. The opposite happened.

NOTE: Here Dr. Farr explains, with diagrams, the following results of his many hydrogen peroxide experiments:

1. The metabolic rate was significantly increased.
2. A stronger concentration would make the metabolic rate go up quicker than weaker ones, but they would both level out to the same rate, due to the body's regulatory enzyme reactions.
3. Mitochondrial action was stimulated, even doubled.
4. Unlike oxygen's properties of contracting the vessels, dilation of the small arteries of the body occurred.
5. The oxygen produced by the H_2O_2 injections did leave the body through the expired air from the lungs, but as it bubbled up, it was re-absorbed.

PEROXIDATION

We're saying: this is not oxygen by itself, that does all these fantastic things. This is something else. This is a peroxidation. The burning up. It's doing a lot of things in metabolism that we don't understand yet. We measured temperature because when you race an engine, it's going to produce heat. The same thing happens in the body. Your temperature goes up, and stays up, while you're being infused with hydrogen peroxide.

SUMMARY OF EXPERIMENTS

This is really what we proved from these experiments: that oxygen doesn't leave the body, it comes out in the lungs and goes back in. That effect, has proven to be extremely beneficial medically.

PULMONARY DISEASE

Have you ever seen someone with chronic pulmonary disease?

They're sick all the time. They can't breathe. They're coughing. They have a terrible life. As a physician, this has been very disheartening because you want to help them so much, but you just don't know what to do. You give them aerosols. You give them the penicillin, and so forth. Try to keep them infection free. Try to keep the lungs as clear as you can, which is not very much, and watch them choke to death.

Let's say a person has chronic pulmonary disease. Those alveoli, those air sacs in the lungs, they're full of all kinds of germs, all kinds of cells, secretions, bacteria, all kinds of things. It's giving them a hard time with living. If this gas comes out and goes back, this is what it might be doing. It may come out in the bottom of the air sacs, underneath the accumulated toxins, undermining that material, and cleaning it out from the bottom up. Wouldn't that be great, to be able to go in there and sweep all that up, and clean it out at one time? Killing the bacteria as it went through there. Then the oxygen goes back in. If that happened, we'd have something like this. Keep somebody breathing until that mucous and everything is cut loose, then they cough it out. That was my idea. In practicality, it works.

Note: This part explained to the author's satisfaction, his own experience with taking hydrogen peroxide for a month, then having a bubbling sensation in the lungs, and coughing up old waste products for 2 months.

We have had several people with chronic obstructive pulmonary disease that we had been treating for years and years. They were hypoxic, no oxygen. They were sick all the time, running a fever because they had constant bacterial infections which we treated with hydrogen peroxide. What happened was this: you hook them up to the hydrogen peroxide. My first one, her name was Cliffie. I had been working with her for several years. I had seen a tremendous breakdown in her health over the past four or five years. She was getting worse, quick. I said: I don't know what this will do to you. It may kill you. Life is not very good the way you are. Let's try it. If you're not afraid, I'm not afraid to give it to you. I've got to prove it to myself. It's a very exciting substance. I wanted to make sure it was safe. I gave it to myself for the first personal test. I didn't want to give myself something to ruin me. I know it's real safe. We started Cliffie on this hydrogen peroxide. Her first treatment. Hooked her up. I walked out of the room.

All of a sudden I heard her gagging and coughing and was sure she was dying. I rushed back in there. She was coughing copious amounts of material out. She couldn't really get her breath. It was just really dramatic. I went over and shut this stuff off. I stopped it from running. The nurses were panicked. They thought she was dying. We shut it off and within about 20 seconds or so, she quit coughing, or slowed back down to her normal cough a minute. I talked to Cliffie and we decided she gagged on something else or maybe it was just one of those things. I turned it back on

again, and she started coughing again. I turned it back off and
she quit. I sat there and played with it. I turned it on, she
would cough. I turned it off, and she would quit. What we were
doing was this: we were emptying her from the bottom up. Cleaning
those lungs out. She said let it run, I can take this. It's OK.
We did.

We sat there while she coughed and coughed and coughed. She
went home, and coughed some more. By the next day, she was feeling
better than she had felt in five years. We have given her a
treatment a week now, for about eight treatments. She is feeling
remarkably better. The chronic diarrhea she had is gone. The
chronic fever she had is gone. She is coughing very little.

Before she could only walk from one chair to the other. Now,
she can get on a trampoline and bounce a little bit. She feels
tremendously better. - Not all the time, when you treat pulmonary
disease, do you get this same "Alka-Seltzer effect". To get this
Alka-Seltzer effect you have to have mucous come out of the
alveoli. Some people have staph infections up in the bronchii. It
doesn't work that way. It gives them oxygen, which is very
important. Part of it gives them oxygen, the peroxide part of it
burns up the toxins, so you are destroying the bacteria. At the
same time we get the mucous loose.

GANGRENE

A gangrenous leg is the wrath of life. A doctor friend of
mine sent me this patient. He said, you've got to do something
soon with this guy, if you can. I have already given him 100
chelation treatments and not much has happened.

Once something is dead and gone, you are not going to bring it
back to life. The decision is this: that leg was dead from a
certain point down. Above that point, we have a zone. We have a
zone that is highly infected, just above that gangrenous area. A
lot of bacteria. We have this blood vessel on the far side. (Here
he illustrates a blood vessel and points out the bacteria and
toxins.) Above that, you have a toxic zone that is neither healthy
or dead. It is kind of in-between. Above that, we have a healthy
zone. Why is this important? For an amputee, it is very
important. If you cut that leg off above the knee, then there are
all kinds of problems in walking, if ever. A prosthesis above the
knee is very difficult to handle. Usually, only young people get
by with those.

What we were hoping for, was an amputation below the knee.
What we did, was give him hydrogen peroxide. Large amounts, every
day. We did it because we knew it would help destroy these toxins,
we knew it would help destroy these bacteria. After about five
days, the toxic zone had gotten lesser. The infected zone had
gotten less. We treated him ten days. It continued down to the
point where we had a sharp demarcation between the gangrene and the
normal healthy tissue. At the tenth day, it was very sharply
demarcated, where it was kind of fuzzy before. He went back to his
doctor. He went into surgery the next day and they did a below the
knee amputation. They said this area up here was as clean as could
be. No toxic areas. No infection. Nothing there. Very, very

clean. We would like to say that we could restore health to that leg, but that's overdone. We did the next best thing. We gave him a below the knee amputation, instead of above the knee. The hydrogen peroxide did this. There is nothing else you can do it with.

ARTERIOSCLEROSIS

Some studies said, if we inject this in the arteries, we know it dissolves triglycerides and cholesterol and takes the plaque out. We thought this action might have a potential effect of reversing arteriosclerosis. It does. (Shows picture) Here is one of a carotid artery going up into the neck. Here is where it was blocked before. They gave peroxide in this artery. There you can see the blood going up into the head. Down here is the leg. You can see that it's partially blocked. Over here it's opened up. Other people have shown that this has dramatic healing effects.

AIDS

Remember what we said about the white cells being able to eat things up? Look here. What they have just come out with, about two weeks ago, in USA Today, "White Blood Cells May Help Block AIDS Virus". We know it does that through the utilization of hydrogen peroxide, in some way.

This information we have learned. We've spread it far and wide, through this article "Intravenous Use of Hydrogen Peroxide". A scientific article. It has already proven to be wonder substance. We have used it in so many different things now. They have given 600 or 700 treatments. That doesn't sound like very many, it really isn't. We've only been doing this for about six months, or less.

FLU

We've found this in someone with the flu. The hard influenza syndrome they're having all over the country now. We had several people come in. Within two days, they are back to work, and completely symptom free.

ASTHMA

We have found that it cures children with asthmatic problems. They had been treated for years and years. We can stop an asthmatic attack within a few hours.

What I want you to be aware of, is that this is something on the rise, and it's going to be very exciting in medicine. It's a whole new way of thinking about medicine. We've always thought of peroxide as something terrible, as harmful, to us. We are finding out that it isn't. We are going to have to change and adjust our thinking, instead of concentrating on vitamin E, vitamin A, and things that are antioxidants, we're going to start using oxidation as a medical tool. It's a whole new area of medicine. Thank you, very much.

- End of Dr. Farr's address.

FARR WRITES NEWSLETTER
PROMOTES FORUMS AND REFERRALS

Dr. Charles Farr is one of the foremost experts in the current H_2O_2 infusion research area. In the IBOM (International Bio-Oxidative Medicine) newsletter, he states: "Any reactions from patients being infused was lessened by pre-infusing the vessel with heparin, but sometimes even after 20 infusions, they might get a reaction." He speculates that, "the infusions, in such cases, might have been too rapid, or the blood flow was reduced." Some of the early literature states they use .15% H_2O_2, but that concentration caused too much cell lysis (decomposition). They now use a 0.0375% level in their therapeutic studies, filtered through a .22 um Millipore Pharmacy Transfer Set, (Cat # IVGS0105S), and advise against using .3% because of possible bubble formation. Patience, is the rule. Some chronic disease patients don't respond for a long time, and need lower dosages paced further apart. The use of antioxidants, like vitamin C, may be counterproductive on the same day of treatment. Note: See section on SOD.

I strongly advise any doctor planning on this oxygenation method, to contact IBOM, for details. Like this: Patients on bronchiodilators may have bubbles passing through pulmonary arteries, so they advise physicians against having both present on the same day, and everyone else should leave this to the doctors to work out. IBOM encourages membership, holds annual conferences, and can be reached at: IBOM, Ozone & Peroxide Referrals, P.O. Box 13205-OT, Oklahoma City, OK 73113, phone 405/478-4266.

IBOM REFERS PEOPLE TO A DOCTOR FROM A LIST OF ABOUT 85 DOCTORS IN THE U.S. THAT GIVE H_2O_2 INTRAVENOUSLY. MANY HAVE TAKEN TRAINING FROM DR. FARR. IT IS CONSIDERED BY THEM TO BE LEGAL - AS IT IS NOT A DRUG, BUT A SUBSTANCE NATURALLY PRODUCED BY THE BODY.

The FDA (as of July 88) has not ruled upon this matter either way. Let's hope they read this book before they do, or at least track down all it's references. The only problems that have shown up are, people using too strong concentrations, or infusing too fast. That's a "people" problem, not an H_2O_2 problem.

MEDICAL REFERENCES ON INFUSING H_2O_2:

1. Balla, G.A., J. W. Finney, and J. T. Mallams: " A method for selective tissue oxygenation utilizing continuous regional intra-arterial infusion technics". Amer. Surg., 29: 496-498, July 1963.

2. Finney, J. W., J. T. Mallams, and G. A. Balla: "Increased available oxygen through regional intra-arterial infusion of dilute hydrogen peroxide". Proc. Amer. Ass. Cancer Res., 3: 318, April 1962.

3. Mallams, J. T., J. W. Finney, and G. A. Balla: "The use of hydrogen peroxide as a source of oxygen in a regional intra-arterial infusion system". Southern Med. Journal, 55: 230-232, 1962.

REFERENCES CAUTIONING ORAL USE OF H_2O_2:

1. Ito A, Watanabe H, Naito M, et al: "Induction of Duodenal Tumors in Mice by Oral Administration of Hydrogen Peroxide". GANN 1981; 72:174-175. Note: There are species differences between humans and mice, and the FDA reviewed this study, and found it to be: "insufficient evidence."

2. Bielski BHJ, Arudi RL, Sutherland MW: "A Study of the Reactivity of H_2O_2/O_2- with Unsaturated Fatty Acids". J. Biol Chem 1983; 258: 4759-4761 Note: Refers to undigested food reacting with H_2O_2.

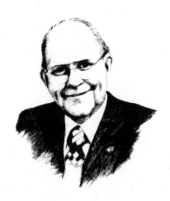

DR. KURT DONSBACH

We now turn to excerpts from a talk given by Dr. Kurt Donsbach, Ph.D.,D.Sc.,N.D.,D.C. He is probably one of the best known alternative health writers, having a selection of his small booklets in just about every health food store. He originally opposed the use of hydrogen peroxide, because it produced "free radicals", which everyone at the time thought was unhealthy. To him, anything that worked on such a basic level sounded too good to be true. After his own wife started taking it, he did his own research, & was amazed at the results - and now advocates it! His organization runs a clinic in Mexico. Dr. Donsbach's talk:

Thank you very much. It is a pleasure to be here. The subject that I am going to address today, requires, that the whole truth be known about it. The half-truth about anything oftentimes does not tell the whole story. I was brought up in a family, in which, truthfulness was highly prized. When I became an adult I tried, on a couple of occasions, to follow those edicts, but only half way. I found out quickly, that half truths get you into all kinds of trouble.

DONSBACH LEARNS ALL RADICALS NOT BAD

Hydrogen peroxide has been alternately labeled as a miracle cure and as a possible inducer of cancer and a number of other conditions, because it might cause free radical damage. I know that this is a concern of many individuals who have heard about it and, therefore, we need to understand, totally, what this hydrogen peroxide is, that has exploded onto the scene in the United States. Very frankly, I have to tell you that for a full year and a half after I first heard about hydrogen peroxide, I discounted it, and perhaps I, personally, was the starting point of most of this misinformation about free radical "bad effects" from the use of hydrogen peroxide. As a result, I have had to eat those words on many occasions. I willingly do so because; once I was put on the proper pathway of learning as to what hydrogen peroxide really is, and what it does, it was a real revelation to me.

49

HYDROGEN AND OXYGEN BALANCE

We should look to the Merck Index, perhaps as a: "Bible of the Chemical Industry," as to just what hydrogen peroxide is. The chemical synonym for hydrogen peroxide is hydrogen dioxide. It is 94% oxygen! It is in this oxygen factor that we really have, in my opinion, the story of hydrogen peroxide. Before we go any further with hydrogen peroxide, let's take a look at oxygen.

When we look at oxygen, we have to understand that there are four basic ingredients that make up our bodies, although there are 70 or so, altogether. The four basic ingredients in the human body are: carbon, nitrogen, hydrogen, and oxygen. We are quite aware that nitrogen is the basic component of the protein part of our body. The protein part of our body is that which, basically, makes up all of our cellular structure. The hydrogen part of this formulation is what solidifies the protein structures. In order to give you an example of why, or how this works, Ill give you an example: the food companies use this concept very well, in that they use hydrogen to convert a very fluid oil, into a very solid substance known as oleo-margarine. They force hydrogen gas literally, into an oil to create a butter substitute, or margarine.

Hydrogen is the solidifying part of our body. We term it anabolic. It builds up the human body, which is good. Oxygen, on the other hand, is catabolic. It tears down, but more important, oxygen cleanses. Oxygen cleans the clinkers out of the furnace. Oxygen destroys the side products, or metabolites, of anabolism, the building up process of the body. We need a proper balance of these two, for the human body to properly function as it should.

DONSBACH EXPLAINS HOW ARTHRITIS IS AFFECTED BY OXYGEN

Many of you have heard that this substance, hydrogen dioxide, or hydrogen peroxide, was originally touted by Walter Grotz because he met Father Willhelm on a cruise ship, and they got to talking, and Wally Grotz was complaining about his arthritis, and Father Willhelm said, "Wally, why don't you try hydrogen peroxide?" Wally tried hydrogen peroxide and, voila, he lost his arthritis in a period of about six weeks. Why? Have you ever heard a person who has arthritis say, "It's going to rain. My knee tells me so."? Why would a person who has arthritis be a weather prophet? As the moisture content of the air increases, we slowly begin to displace the oxygen content of the air with a different substance, H_2O, which has more hydrogen than oxygen. This decrease the oxygen concentration. Arthritis depends upon our ability to mobilize, and clear out, the clinkers in the cells, in order for it not to be activated. We have, in the atmosphere we breathe, a lessening of the ingredient necessary to do so; oxygen; and so the individual hurts.

Oftentimes, the individual is told to go to a dry climate. Also, preferably, not high up in the mountains, but lower, to sea level. Something like Phoenix, Arizona, or Tucson, Arizona. Many times, individuals who go to those hot dry climates, get relief from their arthritis. It isn't cured, but they have less aggravating times. As you get closer to sea level, you also have a higher concentration of oxygen. As you get higher up, you have a

50

lesser concentration of oxygen. The air becomes, "thin". Less oxygen concentration. People who have arthritic type disorders, don't do as well in high altitude as they do at lower altitudes. Again, because of the lack of oxygen. I hope I have brought to you a little bit of the reason why oxygen is so important to the physiology of the human body... to get rid of waste products. Many of you have seen hydrogen peroxide applied to wounds. What happens? It foams and gives all kinds of activity signs. The oxygen that is trapped in the hydrogen peroxide molecule is released, in contact with bacteria. You have what is called an oxidative reaction. The bacteria is destroyed by this oxidative reaction. Infection doesn't occur.

When I first began studying hydrogen peroxide, I didn't really know all these things. I think I've been about as well educated in many respects in chemistry and biochemistry and physiology, and so forth, as most individuals, but these things about hydrogen peroxide totally escaped me, as I think it does most individuals today who have misconceptions about hydrogen peroxide.

H_2O_2 NATURALLY PRODUCED IN BODY

I did not know, as an example, that one of the major defense systems in the human body gives us hydrogen peroxide. Your cells produce hydrogen peroxide all the time. There is, in fact, a part of the cell called a peroxisome, whose job is to produce hydrogen peroxide in order to get rid of viruses and bacteria and other contaminating substances that might get into the cell. The peroxisome literally causes the bacteria to disintegrate, or, explode.

CANDIDA

That kind of knowledge, or half knowledge, led to the concern that many people had. That if one were to use hydrogen peroxide intravenously, it would cause what is called a gas emboli, which would potentially be fatal to the individual. I began to use hydrogen peroxide as a treatment for a now very prevalent epidemic in the civilized countries of the world, candidiasis, because I had been totally frustrated with all of the approaches to candidiasis. The Mystatin-type approach, and we can go on and on to the herbs, and the dietary approaches, to the care of candidiasis. I'll tell you right now, without any fear of valid' contradiction, diet doesn't cause candidiasis, diet will not cure candidiasis. That is statement number 1. Statement number 2, is: the anti-fungal, anti-yeast, preparations, (the drugs, that are commonly used to kill candida) only work in the gut. Their characteristic is that they are not well absorbed into the bloodstream and that is why they are effective in destroying Candida in the gut. Candida in the gut doesn't really bother individuals to any great extent. We all have Candida in the gut. It's only when that Candida migrates through a tear in the gut wall, or through some other orifice, that it gets internally into the systemic portion of the anatomy. Then we begin to have the emotional or mental symptoms of candidiasis. We begin to have the adult onset of allergies that are so significant of - and indicative of - candidiasis.

The things that are occurring, are occurring inside the body. Not, in that closed tube of the gut. The things that are presently being used to control candidiasis are, in whole, basically ineffective.

INTRAVENOUS H_2O_2

The use of hydrogen peroxide intravenously, has been an absolute revelation to me in that we can predict, in 21 days, a total freedom of candidiasis systemically in an individual who has it. We went so far as to guarantee the total freedom from candidiasis in 21 days at our hospital, in Mexico, after the treatment. We can prove that it's there when you come, we can prove it's gone when you leave. I was enormously pleased. It felt like we were really doing something. But, I noticed that some of my Candida patients also had other problems that appeared to be relieved by the use of intravenous hydrogen peroxide. The first time I used intravenous hydrogen peroxide, I was scared out of my skull. Why? Because no one had used it in modern day history intravenously. In 1920 some doctors in India had infused it in terminally ill patients and it had fabulous results. Modern day medicine has not been using hydrogen peroxide. I picked a patient I didn't think would sue me, myself. I started infusing hydrogen peroxide. That's why I was so damn scared, too. I want to tell you, other than the thumping of my heart, nothing really happened. I didn't fall over dead. I had three MD's standing waiting with poised needles to resuscitate me. Nothing happened.

We began using it in ever increasing dosages to find out what the base tolerant level is. We found that there is a certain level that, if you go over it, doesn't do any good at all, not that it does any harm, but it doesn't do any good. Note: Powerful oxidizers can burn you. Leave this experimentation to the M.D.'s.

DONSBACH EXPERIMENTS ON CANCER

We started using it in other conditions of the human body. I think one of the most dramatic, was work with cancer patients. When you have a clinic in Mexico, you never see noncritical cancer patients. You only see the patients that every doctor has given up on, that has been surgically butchered, that has been chemically destroyed and radiated and burned sometimes beyond recognition. I have seen individuals who have had their bowels fused with scar tissue from radiation, who have had their total immune system a lymph count of 5 or less when they come down to see us. We began to see these people turning around. To get a 10% or 20% cure rate on patients like that is really quite good. To get the kind of results we started to see, was unbelievable. I didn't publish them, I didn't talk about them for quite some time. I knew the bubble had to break. I knew there had to be something that would come in that would destroy the elation I felt with what I was seeing. I want to put a caveat in here, right now.

We use a great deal more than just hydrogen peroxide in our approach to cancer, as well as all the other chronic degenerative diseases that we treat. It is my opinion that hydrogen peroxide, because of its great oxidative action, will assist the human body in destroying a cancer cell.

Remember, according to Warburg and others, that cancer cells are anaerobic. They function without oxygen. They are not an oxygen-loving cell. Oxygen destroys anaerobic bacteria and anaerobic cells.

BLOOD COLOR CHANGES, PATIENTS FEEL "CLEARER"

We can prove with blood samples that we can hyperoxygenate your bloodstream better with hydrogen peroxide than by breathing oxygen. Better than by infusing ozone, which we used to do, either rectally or into the bloodstream directly. Better than by putting the patient into a hyperbaric oxygen chamber. We can increase the oxygenation level in the body tremendously. You can see the difference, in the color of the blood, of a patient who has had hydrogen peroxide infused into them. Oftentimes, if you've ever seen a person who is not well cut themselves, the blood has a dark bluish, purplish color that is obviously not healthy. When you start infusing hydrogen peroxide, the blood we draw when we take samples, is a bright, healthy, red color that looks good. I'm not saying that there still aren't things wrong with it, but we know it has a basic good oxygen content because we've tested it, and others have tested it, and we know that we can oxygenate this blood.

Oftentimes, patients tell us, "I feel so much clearer. It's funny to say, I feel clearer." When you start oxidating toxins in the human body and destroying those clinkers in the furnace, sure you're going to feel lighter and freer. Patients tell me, "My head is clearer. I'm thinking clearer. I can stay on a subject longer; before, I wandered very easily. I couldn't concentrate, now I can."

DONSBACH DISCOVERS H_2O_2 EASES TRANSITION TO DEATH

We don't save all our patients, and I think that none of us likes to see death or be with death. I don't know that any doctor ever gets used to the death that is a part of the practice of healing. I can tell you that we get so many of these patients who are brought in with medical ambulances, air ambulances, and on stretchers. Many of those we see die, because they are practically dead when they come. After the infusion of hydrogen peroxide, there is often a peace that comes over them. There is a lack of pain. There is a lack of confusion. Many times you'll see persons who came in, fighting everything, fighting their family, fighting therapy and so forth, who now relax and accept what's happening and pass away in peace. That, at least, is to some extent, a benefit that I had never seen before, when I had seen and observed death. It is a privilege to be able to help in that way.

PEOPLE USE H_2O_2 ORALLY

Many people have used hydrogen peroxide orally. I have been asked many, many times: "Doesn't it form hydroxyl groups in the stomach and cause cancer of the stomach?" Father Willhelm, of course, has a lot more years of experience, of watching individuals drink hydrogen peroxide, than I have. I do know of some valid experiments done where rather copious quantities of hydrogen peroxide were caused to be ingested by animals. There is no evidence of any hydroxyl formation in animal stomachs. They use animals that are similar to man in their chemistry and in their physiology in order to do this.

Research is a great teacher. It is also the field of a lot of people who use facts to prove their theories. I remember very clearly a famous professor telling me when I was going to school: "If you only have to throw out half the facts to prove your theory, the research is a success." Oftentimes that's what happens in research. Somebody is trying to prove something and he throws out those facts that occur, that are contradictory, and keeps those that are complimentary.

I feel very, very confident knowing this much;, that there are a couple of caveats, and maybe you should all wake up now just for a moment, if you're going to drink hydrogen peroxide. Drink it on an empty stomach. Allow as little reactivity as you can in the stomach so as much can be absorbed as possible. If you have a lot of food in there, the bacteria in that food is going to react with the hydrogen peroxide. You're going to have foaming and the possibility is you're going to vomit. Then you're going to say, how can you possibly get me to drink something that causes me to vomit.

That's the first thing that happened to me when I went down, full of fire, to try hydrogen peroxide on my sick patients at the hospital. I had sick patients who were vomiting all over the place and threatening mutiny and telling me, if I ever came close to them with another drink of hydrogen peroxide, I'd get a swift kick, you know where.

I began to work with that problem a little bit and we found that; by taking hydrogen peroxide and putting it in a base of aloe vera, which also is very pure in that it doesn't allow bacteria in its presence, but has a carminative or stomach settling effect, that we could tolerate it much more. I then became a little more crafty and I added lemon flavoring and berry flavoring and herbal tea flavoring to let the mouth know that it was good. We were soon giving it away at conventions, such as this. I had people coming up and coming back and saying give me another shot and drinking this stuff, not knowing that they were drinking hydrogen peroxide, but thinking they were drinking flavored aloe vera. Some of them complained that there was a mild nausea later on. They were wondering what they ate, never dreaming it was the hydrogen peroxide that they had taken. It is very tolerable in that type of circumstance.

EXPERIMENTS SHOW H$_2$O$_2$ RELIEVED PAIN OF INFUSIONS

More important, perhaps, is that you can use it in many different ways. We found it had pain-relieving qualities. I don't know how many of you have ever had intravenous infusion. How many - while you were having infusions - had pain in the arm and the vein, and so forth? I found that by rubbing hydrogen peroxide diluted on that area we could relieve the pain in something like 3 to 4 seconds. Amazing!

BUNIONS, MOUTH DISEASE, SINUSES, COLDS

So, I tried it on a variety of things. Bunions. It has pain-relieving qualities that are really amazing, so we formulated a pain gel. It's great for pyorrhea, to prevent dental plaque, to prevent mouth conditions that cause bad breath and all these other associated things. Soft spongy gums. Tooth gel that you can brush your teeth with. Nasal spray for the sinuses. If you want to go to a movie and cry, the best thing to do is take a little shot of this nasal spray of hydrogen peroxide, the tears flow. Just in a few seconds, so do the sinuses. The sinuses open up like you've never known and you're expectorating mucous, oftentimes so foul smelling that now you know why people backed off when you were talking to them. Many of us have pockets of infection in those sinuses that are never touched by anything that we used. We scrub our outside, but how do you scrub your sinuses? The possibilities are literally endless. A gargle for sore throats that will stop a cold literally in its tracks. How many of you can tell when you're going to get a cold by that little tickle in the top part of your throat, at your nasopharynx? If you'll gargle and spray with hydrogen peroxide, that's the end of those viruses. They're gone. They can't multiply anymore. So the use of hydrogen peroxide is literally endless. They are so many things we can do with it.

DONSBACH'S WIFE CHANGES HIS SKEPTICISM

I just don't know how to thank, first, Father Willhelm; second, Wally Grotz; third, my wife who heard Father Willhelm and Wally Grotz. I didn't listen. I heard the lecture, but I didn't listen. I was sitting back there in my own cloud, knowing when I heard Father Willhelm say that the hydrogen peroxide came down in rainwater and I just turned the channel. I wasn't listening. My wife listened and she came home and said:

"I heard you say that hydrogen peroxide wasn't good."

I said "Yes, It forms free radicals and causes all kinds of problems."

She said, "Well, I'm going to try it."

I said, "You didn't hear me!"

She said, "Yes, I did; but I also heard them. Maybe they're smarter than you are?"

LACK OF PROFIT HAS SLOWED COMMERCIAL DEVELOPMENT

If there was any way to get my attention, she found the way. That was when I called Wally Grotz and said, "You claim to have some literature that documents hydrogen peroxide." Wally Grotz sent me a stack of literature, that he had accumulated from studies. That was my beginning with hydrogen peroxide. Maybe you really ought to thank my wife. That's how I began. It is absolutely amazing, the amount of work that has been done with this simple substance. I think that Father Willhelm sums it up greatly when he said; he went to a major drug company trying to get them to do what we have done; to put out products with hydrogen peroxide as basic over-the-counter remedies, for a number of things. The man at that drug company said, "Father Willhelm, we know about hydrogen peroxide, but, frankly speaking, we are a profit motivated company and there is no profit in hydrogen peroxide." Unfortunately, that may be the reason that hydrogen peroxide has been the sleeper in the medical field that it really is. Because I don't know of anything that has the broad spectrum applications that this particular product has in everyday life.

H_2O_2 USED IN BATHS

We use it in our jacuzzis, we put patients in there with 48 ounces of hydrogen peroxide in the water. I have seen an arthritic knee, locked up tight, get approximately 80% motion in less than two weeks after external use of hydrogen peroxide. How much did it cost? Less than $5.00 worth of hydrogen peroxide. If you can do something like that, how can you call that profit oriented quackery? It isn't. It is something that all of us can make use of, and some of you may wish to.

DONSBACH RESPONDS TO AUDIENCE QUESTIONS

I know this is a controversial and new subject, I would like to answer questions on it, rather than talking about what I want to talk about.

Q. Are you saying that by juicing fruits or vegetables, that we are releasing hydrogen peroxide? I would say; from what I know of chemistry and so forth, no, that's not true. Activating hydrogen peroxide literally deactivates it. On contact with other substances, it readily breaks down into water and oxygen and that oxygen is quickly dispersed in seconds. When we infuse it into the body, the reason it doesn't immediately separate into water and oxygen, is; there is a substance called cytochrome-C that slows that down, and literally preserves it. That's, perhaps, why the body manufactures cytochrome-C. To preserve hydrogen peroxide intact in the body. We can preserve infused hydrogen peroxide in the body measurably up to 30 to 40 minutes after infusion. That is a protectant. But, when you juice something, you're literally tearing it apart, and would be opening up that bond and creating oxygen which might float off as a gas, or be otherwise combined very quickly in the juice, long before you could drink it.

Q. I use it as an antibiotic. Would I use it as an enema? Be very careful when you use hydrogen peroxide as an enema, or in a colonic. It is grossly powerful stuff. It will clean the entire gut of mucous membranes if you use too much. It is fantastic. It will break up impactions and everything else.

CAUTIONS ON STRENGTH OF SOLUTION

Perhaps before I answer any other questions, let's be sure of what I am talking about. I am not talking about, at this point, drug store variety hydrogen peroxide. Throughout my whole talk, when I spoke of hydrogen peroxide, I was speaking about what is known as 35% food grade hydrogen peroxide. Diluted to a dosage or strength of less than: 1 & 1/2%, oftentimes, down to as little as .075%, or less.

COLONICS

When I use it in colonics, in the clinic, we put the equivalent of approximately 10 drops of pure 35% hydrogen peroxide in five gallons of water. That's pretty dilute, but it does some remarkable things at that dilution.

H_2O_2 LEGAL AS FOOD PRESERVATIVE WORLDWIDE

Hydrogen peroxide has been accepted by the food and drug commissions around the world, as a preservative. As an example; have you ever bought the juices off the shelf that are just in a cardboard container, and they never go bad on you? Do you know what preserves them? Hydrogen peroxide. In Europe, the shelf life of milk is kept for as along as three and four weeks, sitting on the shelf without refrigeration, by using hydrogen peroxide. I do not believe they can ban or outlaw hydrogen peroxide. We may have to play with the labeling. You say, they could classify it as a drug? Sure, maybe. It is classified, technically, as a food or as a food additive, all over the world. It would take some major changing, I believe, to do that. There are a number of things, because of the simplicity of the compound; there may be ways of bootlegging it.

Q. How much would you use at one time? Good question. I should address it. There are individuals who have used, it in very low dosages, such as one or two drops, two or three times a day. Remember, on an empty stomach. That means, three hours after eating, and 20 minutes before eating. We tell patients; take it on arising and at bedtime. When you get up in the morning and when you go to bed at night. That is, so you can feel bad all day, and all night. (laughter).

DONSBACH STATES HIS DOSAGE

Remarkably though, I have had thousands of people who have called me and said how much better they have felt, once they started using this, for any number of conditions. My suggested therapeutic maintenance dosage is 25 drops (of the 35% food grade, diluted by putting it in a glass of water, before you drink it.), twice a day. However, many people do very well on 10 drops, twice a day, or 15 drops twice a day. My cancer patients, ONLY if they are in active cancer, I put them on 75 drops, twice a day, of 35% food grade hydrogen peroxide. We dilute that, obviously.

NOTE: IF 35% HYDROGEN PEROXIDE IS NOT DILUTED, IT WILL BURN YOU ANYWHERE IT TOUCHES YOUR BODY! ALSO NOTICE, THAT MANY ADVOCATE USING IT SPARINGLY, UNLESS YOU HAVE AN ACTUAL ILLNESS.

Q. You are not clear on how much you are supposed to take? I think the biggest confusion, is about percentages. Totally forget about percentages. It is quantity that counts. 35% food grade hydrogen peroxide: anywhere, from one, two, up to, in acute cases, 75 drops twice a day. (NOTE: Most people interviewed by the author only went up to 25 drops, 2 or 3 times a day) From one to 75 drops, twice a day. Preferably staying in the lower half of that area.

Q. How large a glass of water? Six to 12 ounces of water or juice. The more drops of H_2O_2, the more dilution you'll want. One or two drops can be put in water and you'll never know the difference. It tastes just a little bit flatter than normal, but other than that, you will have no change in flavor. Of course, the higher you get, the more change you will have.

DONSBACH METHODS OF REMOVING UNPLEASANT TASTE

You can put it, as I said, in aloe vera to make it a little more palatable. There are a number of things. Cinnamon seems to hide the aftertaste that people have. Some non-sugared cinnamon chewing gum afterwards will often take away the effervescing aroma that sticks to your mouth after you take it. You should find something that is non-food, such as chewing gum, temporarily. Chewing tobacco will take it out also, but I don't recommend it.

DOES IT HARM FRIENDLY BACTERIA?

Q. Isn't there a problem of destroying beneficial bacteria if you're going to take hydrogen peroxide on a daily basis? Excellent question. The beneficial bacteria in the human gut, are aerobic, not anaerobic. Therefore, they love oxygen and will thrive on hydrogen peroxide.

SIDE EFFECTS

Q. Do you have any side effects while you're getting better? I think the biggest side effect is that for some people, if they start too fast, the elimination of toxins overwhelms their liver and kidneys and they temporarily feel worse, rather than better. I tell them, you have two choices: 1) back off your dosage by half increments until you're not feeling that way, or, 2) accept the fact that this is what's happening, just pour the water and herb teas to yourself, and grit your teeth and go on. It won't last too long, a few days at most. As far as serious side effects, no. If I wish to mix it in a nasal spray, it is kind of touchy. The nasal mucosa is extraordinarily sensitive. As you know, by just breathing some things, you sneeze and so forth. I have to be careful to get a physiological saline solution to put this in, then I mix it with some glycerin and some other things. The product is commercially available.

58

Q. Will the use of hydrogen peroxide in an enema bag stimulate the liver to throw out the poisons that are in the liver? I would not count on that. Let me explain something: the liver would be very, very happy, to throw out the toxins that are accumulated within the liver, the moment you start detoxifying the rest of the body. The liver will accumulate toxins only when the eliminative channels are not adequate to get rid of what is in the blood, and the kidneys, primarily, purify the blood. So it will begin to accumulate these toxins, holding them free from the bloodstream.

DONSBACH TREATED CANDIDA

I tell ladies how to clean the vaginal tract with a weak dilution of hydrogen peroxide, because it will clean up candidiasis totally in that area. Whether it makes you feel that much better, I am unwilling to say.

PARKINSON'S

Q. Does it have a beneficial effect on a disease such as Parkinson's Disease? I don't know. We have treated several Parkinson's patients. In order to separate the wheat from the chaff, all of my patients get hydrogen peroxide. I don't care if they come in for nosebleeds or whatever, they get hydrogen peroxide. My Parkinson's patients get a lot of other therapy, including live- cell therapy, which we feel has a beneficial effect on Parkinson's Disease. To give the credit to hydrogen peroxide, is not fair.

EPSTEIN-BARR VIRUS

Q. How does it help chronic Epstein-Barr virus? I know that we can solve the Epstein-Barr situation, but I do not believe we can solve it with hydrogen peroxide alone. I use an anti-viral compound which is illegal in the United States and Canada, called Riboverin. It has no side effects and is a fabulous medication that will, in a period of six months, clear up Epstein-Barr. It will not do it overnight, but it will do it in six months. We had an airline pilot who had a very positive Epstein-Barr situation. He was in danger of losing his license. He came to us. He is now Epstein-Barr free, and is a totally different person. He doesn't know himself. It is a very exciting area for those people who have Epstein-Barr.

Note: Father Willhelm has a friend, Fr. Richard Bain, at Saint Thomas Church, in San Francisco, who says he got rid of his Epstein-Barr virus in 3 weeks with the use of hydrogen peroxide.

EMPHYSEMA

Q. Does hydrogen peroxide have any helpful effect on emphysema? I will give you, in 30 seconds, a 20% benefit to all emphysemics. One ounce of 35% hydrogen peroxide (per gallon of water) in a vaporizer every night in an emphysemics bedroom, and they will breathe freer than they have breathed in years! I do this for my lung cancer patients. Patients who could not lie down

in bed to sleep can lie down after one night of breathing the
vapors of hydrogen peroxide. It's amazing. One ounce per gallon.
It's a very simple thing to do.

KIDNEYS

Q. If you have poor kidney function, will hydrogen peroxide be
dangerous? Absolutely not. It will, in fact, help restore kidney
function because you're helping get the clinkers out of the system.
You're detoxifying. Here is where nutrition comes in very
strongly. A while ago, I said: "Bad nutrition didn't cause
candidiasis, therefore nutrition won't cure it." But, nutrition
will help the body be strong enough to overcome a lot of the other
conditions that associate themselves with some of these situations.

TAP WATER

Q. Will tap water be made completely clear by the use of
hydrogen peroxide? It will destroy all of the bacteria. But, it
will not take out the pesticides. It will not take out the
fluoride. We are not promoting hydrogen peroxide as an answer to
purifying water. It will destroy all the bacteria. It will do
that better than chlorine will, without any damage to the body.
There are other contaminants in the stuff we call water. This is
not H2O anymore. It is H2O plus a chemical soup. There are other
things you have to do: put a good filtration system in your home,
take the rest of the crap out, buy purified water. Those are your
choices.

RESEARCH SHOWS FLUORIDE SLOWS OXYGEN UPTAKE

Let me read you something: recently, Russian investigators
have found that fluoride added to our drinking water slows down
the process of burning food, called, "oxidation". The level of
adenotriphosphates is lowered because of fluoride. When the body
burns food, it stores the energy in a substance called ATP, or
adenotriphosphates. During fluoride intoxication, it is reported
that rats and mice have decreased oxygen uptake, reduced expiration
(meaning less carbon dioxide going out), and decreased activities
of oxidation reduction enzymes in the liver and lungs. By the
third month, 31-40% decreases in ATP levels were observed in all
organs. Differences in the responses of red blood cells, liver,
muscle, and brain, were observed after 30 days. What does that
mean? If you've been drinking fluoridated water for a period of
time, you are going to have less oxidative reactions. Therefore
more disease of all kinds - and less energy to fight it with.
Don't drink fluoridated water.

WHERE IS IT LEGAL?

Q. Who is allowed, in the United States, to administer
intravenous hydrogen peroxide? I will preface that by saying, I
took my practice to Mexico. Only those doctors who are crazy
enough to believe they won't be found out, are administering it.
Many doctors come down and stay at our hospital for a couple of
days, get the protocols, go back home, and do it. They don't tell
their patients. They don't tell their staff. They don't tell
their wives. They do it in total secrecy. That's a fact. I wish

we had a dozen doctors in this audience who would be willing to administer it up here. If they were here, I would immediately give them all of the things I have learned about this. People power is the only thing that will ever change the practice of medicine in whatever country it is. If you make yourself heard loud enough, you can change the progress of medical history. It takes you to make changes. You've got to take the time to write letters. You've got to take the time to come to meetings and let your voice be heard. Otherwise, forget it.

It's up to you. It isn't up to us.

Note: This ends Dr. Donsbach's talk, and the "quoted speeches" section of the book.

DR. DONSBACH'S OFFERINGS

Dr. Donsbach has published a 25 page booklet called "Hydrogen Peroxide - H202". His organization runs Hospital Santa Monica, in Rosarito Beach, Mexico, "The largest wholistic hospital in the world". Dr. Donsbach, 323-OT San Ysidro Blvd, San Ysidro, CA, 92073

METHODS OF PEROXIDE PRODUCTION

1. Chemically: - Treat Barium Peroxide with Sulfuric Acid. The Barium Sulfate settles to the bottom and Hydrogen Peroxide is drained off. (To concentrate; it is vacuum distilled.)

2. Treat water with ultraviolet light.

3. Electricity; - silent, or open spark methods.

4. Bubble Ozone (O3) through cold water.

"SUCCESS STORY" PEOPLE INTERVIEWED

Starting with this section, we move away from the talks delivered by the current hydrogen peroxide pioneers, and look into explaining a little more about the history, and workings of our oxygenation subjects.

When someone orders the starter information packet from Walter Grotz's E.C.H.O. (Educational Concerns for Hydrogen & Oxygen, a nonprofit organization), included in it is a list of "H_2O_2 Success Stories". In the spring of 1988, I got in touch with some of those listed. Some were over 70, and had been on H_2O_2 for over 5 years. Here are some excerpts from our discussions, keep in mind most came to oxygenation **after** disease had done a lot of damage. Wisdom dictates living to prevent disease first, not last.

ARTHRITIS

Elke Olson   Braham, Minnesota,

How long did you take H_2O_2? "Since 1982."

Have you noticed any side effects? "You don't get hooked on the stuff. I wouldn't mind dropping it, if I could. It is not the most pleasant-tasting stuff. When something works you don't give it up. I got a severe case of psoriatic arthritis.. took gold shots, Motrin, and had reactions to them all... only could take coated aspirins. My husband came home, & spoke of a guy at work who's arthritis was helped by H_2O_2. My husband wanted me to try it, I was skeptical, since nothing else worked, but I tried it anyway. Took the drugstore Parke Davis brand, started with 1 oz. in 5 oz. of water, next day 2 oz. third day 3 oz... up to 5 oz., three times per day. Couldn't keep it down if I took over 3 oz., so I stayed at 3 oz.... I went to Germany, and my friends made fun of it, I stopped, but it started to hurt again.. Came home & took it in earnest. Took two weeks to get better. Before taking this, I wasn't even able to get up our 15 steps from the basement, in one try. Now I get up and don't have too much trouble with that. Now taking 35% food grade peroxide. Still do get some bad days...humid or cold, but I can live with it. Considering my other alternatives I wouldn't even consider giving it up totally. Now taking 15 drops, once a day... equal to 3 oz. in 5 oz. of water. Also using it on psoriasis lesions."

Hilde Vieau   Delano, Minnesota

"I had rheumatoid arthritis in both my inflamed, swollen, and stiff knees. 2 Cortisone shots didn't help... I was taking pain pills... couldn't stand long... I had a hard time up & down steps... constant pain... one was much worse than the other."

"I met Walter Grotz. Started on a few drops, and worked up to taking the peroxide for almost 4 months, up to 75 drops a day. 25 drops, three times a day. Lucky it didn't upset my stomach . Didn't like it, but took it anyway. It took a long time, about 3 months, before I started showing any improvement, but when it got

62

going it improved fast. Took it for 6 more weeks, tapered off, and by that time I was completely cured. And I haven't had any recurrence."

Did it go away? "Yes. That was 10 years ago. My knees are OK. I have arthritis in the morning. I'm stiff, but I'm 75 years old so I can't expect to feel perfect. I get over it after a little exercise and I'm fine."

ASTHMA & ULCERS

R & J B. (Withheld, their request) Rice Lake, Wisconsin

"I get heartburn as a side effect. Lasts only a short time, an hour at the very most. I've noticed, in talking with people, that you would get heartburn. The oxygen that is in your body is working. I had migraine headaches also with my asthma. When I first started taking peroxide, I started getting absolutely terrific headaches, that I could hardly stand. I cut back on the dosage that I was taking and took it at a slower pace. That's what I did, and the headaches subsided, and they weren't as severe. Pretty soon, I didn't have any headaches. On it for 5 years."

"On my asthma. At first, it cut down and was almost completely gone in a short time. I'd say in a matter of two weeks I had cut down on my medication, and in a month I was not taking it at all. It was wonderful! After I had not been taking it for a year, I got a bad illness... almost like a virus. That set me back. I got asthma all over again. I started on the peroxide three times a day, and I had a hard time for a good three months. After that three months was over, I was like a new person. I haven't had a bit of asthma since. I have heard some people say that you've got to take it in strong doses and really knock it out of you and you'll be sick during that time. It's just like if you had surgery and you have a recuperating time. You feel miserable after surgery. It is just kind of the same thing. It is cleaning out your system."

"If you keep putting bad stuff in your system, again, you're defeating your purpose. That was one thing we could do. Change our diet, and watch what we were eating, and cut down on our food intake also. There were plenty of times I took the peroxide and I just had to sit in the chair and say I do not feel well. I just had to make up my mind. I allowed myself about an hour after I took the peroxide to just sit back and relax and let that oxygen do its work. My husband reacts differently. He has to go out and work. Go out and move around. I can't do that."

What happens when he doesn't move around? "That's just how he feels. He has to go out and move around and get that oxygen through his body, then it works better for him. For me, it's almost like over-stimulation. It's working too hard in my body. Then I don't feel well. Not exactly nauseated, but just kind of ...oh, not feeling good. Like I know something is wrong. If I just sit still, I'm fine. I get up early in the morning and take my peroxide, and I crawl back into bed and read for awhile. We all learn our little methods of how to cope with these things."

"When my husband and I started out on this, we started out on the 3% from the grocery store. 35% was not available to us. If you think 35% is bad to take, just try 3% sometime. You just have to stand there, with the glass in your hand, and say; this is going to do me good. I'm going to take it. I've had asthma all my life. After you go to the doctor and he gives you all these different pills to take, nothing really helps. This doctor said that he believes in preventive medicine. I said that's fine. Let's find out what it is that's causing my asthma. He couldn't do anything for me there, and kept giving me some other kinds of pills and saying: "Try this for two weeks and come back, and, try this for two weeks and come back." Finally, I brought back all the samples he gave me and said: "I don't want any of those anymore. I'll go home and take care of myself." Right after that, about two months later, I met Walter Grotz."

Where did you hear about it before Walter? "We didn't. My husband was at a different meeting, of a different category completely, and at intermission Walter happened to be standing there talking to someone about it, and my husband was right there. He said, "Gosh, this sounds interesting!" He asked if he could listen in. Of course, Walter invited him in. When he came home he was so enthused about it. He said, I know this is the right thing for us to take. So we got on it right away. It's a Godsend. He has been helping us along ever since. I feel that this is a natural thing. This is so much better than man-made things."

CANDIDA

Dorothy Iverson   Mayer, Minnesota.

"I've written an article about my success story. It was published in 1985, in "Health Consciousness Magazine". It has been republished 6 or 8 times, in other magazines, since then. I constantly get requests from people all over the country on how to help them with their problems of Candida."

Was it completely eradicated? "Yes. I'm perfectly well. For some people, just taking it orally doesn't do it for them. I feel that it's not just the peroxide. You have to start a very strenuous nutritional program. You've got to know how to get your body to start digesting and assimilating your food. That's the main problem with Candida, that they're not digesting what they eat. They are not assimilating what they digest, if, they can digest it even. (Note: At first reading, this seems to contradict what Dr. Donsbach said, about nutrition not causing candidiasis, but she is making a different point. She is pointing out the necessity of reestablishing a good immune system through proper nutrition.) I try to help them with diet and supplements. Like I say, peroxide is only half of it. If you just take peroxide and don't do anything about the nutritional part, then you're not going to get well. There's more to it than just the peroxide."

"I was going to a chiropractor for 20 years, for allergies I didn't know I had, that were causing my back problem. After I got the Candida cleared up, then the allergies cleared up, and I don't have to go anymore. I have been answering letters for three years, wondering when is this going to die down."

64

What about the side effects of hydrogen peroxide? "I can't say I've heard of anyone with side effects. You do get nausea from the peroxide. You may get some cleansing reactions. There is a new peroxide gel out that we feel is working real well. (Note: Peroxy gels are reviewed near the end of this book.) You rub it on the skin. You don't take it orally. It is absorbed through the skin. Apparently, there is no nausea from taking it that way. They claim a teaspoonful is equal to 20 drops of hydrogen peroxide. A bottle of it goes for 96 treatments... which is about $15. That is not too high a price. We are going to try that also, on my sister-in-law when she gets back here."

DIABETES

C. F. Dickinson   North Dakota

Can you tell me what it has done for you? "It has helped with the diabetes quite a bit."

Has it stopped the diabetes completely? "No. It is controlled by diet."

How has it helped you? "My diabetes is not so high. I put 5 oz. (3%) in a quart of water. I take 5 oz. in the morning and 5 oz. at night. I had a stroke, so I started taking it."

How long have you been taking the hydrogen peroxide? "About 6 years. My wife takes it for arthritis. She takes it everyday."

Is your wife there? Can I talk to her about her arthritis?
"Mrs. Dickinson: I take the straight Parke-Davis brand. I take 2 teaspoons of peroxide in about 3/4 glass of water. Straight water. That's the way I do it."

How has it helped your arthritis? "I still get a little arthritis. You can't knock it out. Nobody can tell me that. Change of weather, maybe something we eat. I would say that. Otherwise, I'm taking care of my husband in a wheelchair. No nurse or nothing. I think I'm doing pretty good. I'm 77, coming 78. I think, myself, I'm doing good, not just all right. I could be a whole lot worse if I hadn't taken it. Maybe I don't take enough of it, but I don't want to overdo it. It's better to underdo a little bit, than to overdo. That's all I can tell you about myself. I Put 2 teaspoons in 3/4 cup of water in the morning before I have breakfast. Right when I get up. I water my houseplants with it. I really see a difference in them. You don't get a cold so much. My husband never even got the flu. My son had the flu and came and ate with us. We didn't get it. I think that's pretty good. You can tell from how you feel that you're doing good."

LUKEMIA

D. M.   Luverne, Minnesota

I'd like to find out what it did for your leukemia. "I haven't got any big success story to tell on my leukemia. It hasn't turned me around or anything, but I feel it has done me a world of good. I don't know where I would be, if it hadn't been for the peroxide. The first thing it did do for me, was clean up my ulcers. I was doctoring ulcers for 5 years and had to be careful what I ate and took pills, liquids, and so forth. In a matter of just a few weeks after I started on the peroxide, they were gone, forgot them, forget about it. That's no small matter. I've been drinking peroxide for about 5 years."

"For the first few years, I could adjust my white count. My white count is off. I have chronic lymphocytic leukemia. My white count is high. For the first few years, I could adjust it by what I did with the peroxide. If I'd get serious and drink a little more peroxide, I could control my white count. I would kind of slump off, like you tend to do, I would think I was doing good and not drink as much peroxide and my next white count would be up. Repeatedly, I have seen that happen. I eat different. I continue to take about 50 drops of peroxide everyday; 25 first thing in the morning, and 25 before I go to bed. I am not being treated by the doctor's methods. I have learned enough that I will not do it that way. My system has got a problem now, why should I take that junk that they are using and destroy it even further. I absolutely won't. I have learned enough about it that there are other things available nowadays that we can do. We've got to take care of ourselves. I take barley greens, colon cleansers, etc. We can't buy our health back from a doctor."

"I was taking 75-100 drops a day and a heavy level of food supplements. I can't say that the food supplements showed any significant improvement. Possibly there was a reaction between the two. It was 100 drops for three months, I should have gotten a significant adjustment on my white count, which I didn't. It was a little bit surprising to me why, but, I believe it was creating a problem with the higher level of vitamins that something didn't work. You would think between the two you would get a terrific adjustment, but it didn't happen. I feel that I can't be without my peroxide. We just don't have colds anymore. You can't ignore those kinds of things. I sure don't miss my ulcers! That was in 1975, they put me in the hospital. I guess I got on the peroxide program about 1 year after Wally Grotz got started with it. I'm lucky enough to be one of his first followers. In just a short while after, I started on the peroxide program, I just forget about the ulcers. Anytime you can cut out drugs, you're definitely ahead."

MULTIPLE SCLEROSIS

Walter Sohasky   Annandale, Virginia

"Ozone and peroxide, as far as I'm concerned, are terrific things! I hadn't had too much experience with ozone, but I've had my blood ozonated once or twice. Of course, that was not enough to tell, but it certainly did not do me any harm. As far as the hydrogen peroxide is concerned;, I've been on it for more than 4 years now."

"I'm 69 now. When I was about 52 years old I started feeling this weakness in my legs and inability to walk. In 1983 a doctor fresh out of Johns-Hopkins said I had Multiple Sclerosis. I had gone through three prestigious clinics; Georgetown University; Mayo Clinic in Rochester, Minnesota; and Lahey - in Boston."

"I had lost control of my bodily functions to a degree before I took the chemotherapy, but it was after it was absolutely hopeless. I had to go in the shower with my clothes on many times because there was no control even though I sat in the kitchen which is only 3-4 feet from the bathroom. I couldn't make it. You just reach a point where it just starts coming. There's no warning. That's when you have to go in the shower with all your clothes on. That is degrading. For about a year after, I couldn't sleep. It would be 3:00, 4:00 or 5:00 in the morning, before I could doze off. I had a problem swallowing and not choking. I had to take all my food with a washdown of water, milk, coffee or tea, whatever I was having. Otherwise I would gag and start choking. I had a pounding in my ears. It sounded like a pile driver in the distance. I asked my children to check it out for me. They said there was no pounding. By self-examination I realized it was my heartbeat that was pounding in my ears."

"To get back to the peroxide: I had given up on it also. I asked my son to get literature at a health food show. I called Walter Grotz. I didn't know him from Adam. I asked him to send me some peroxide. He sent me 2 quarts without a bill. That floored me right off the bat. I told him I didn't want charity. He said send a donation to ECHO then. That's all he asked. Not for himself, but for ECHO."

"It took about 8 months on the peroxide. I almost gave up on it. I thought it was a hoax. Low and behold, as I say, about 8 months after, I started getting control of my bodily functions. That was worth a million dollars to me. About 8 months after, I started improving, and now I swear - I can go any place. I even went to Dr. Neiper's clinic in Hanover, West Germany. You've heard of him, haven't you? After Neiper's clinic, two weeks there, I went to Munich for other tests. On the way back I did not eat or drink, I was 11 1/2 hours until I was in my home before I went to the bathroom - once. That is amazing, considering I had to live by the bathroom door."

Has it done anything since then? "I'm 69, I'll be 70 in November. It has kept me mentally alert. It has kept me walking around the house with a walker. When I go out, I have to go in a wheelchair. In the house I just use a walker. When I go down to the rec. room I don't even take my walker with me. As long as I have a table or chair or something to hold on to, I can make my way around. I know darn well if it wasn't for the peroxide, I'd be a lot worse off. In my case, my mental ability right now has jumped from where it used to be. It has improved."

How do you think it affects multiple sclerosis, what does it do to clean it up? "I don't think it will clear up multiple sclerosis. I'm being very honest with you because Walter Grotz has been monitoring my condition. I'll tell you, it's certainly keeping me from getting worse. Some MS people even die from the disease. But, in my case I'm mentally alert, and physically I'm alert. The other thing too, is that I had bursitis in my right shoulder to where if I extended my arm, I could only get it to the horizontal position with pain. Now I can point it at the ceiling and do anything I want to. Even with Walter Grotz, he cured his own arthritis with peroxide only. When you've been behind the 8 ball and come out, you're grateful. In fact, that's why I'm dedicating the rest of my life to this, it's costing money. I'm not making anything out of this. I'm spreading the word to the best of my ability, as far as the peroxide is concerned."

"I'm still on it. I'm now taking this aloe vera tonic from Dr. Donsbach's clinic. I like the "cherry-berry" flavor. I've been on that for months. I finally got to the point I could not take the regular peroxide anymore because of the taste and smell. What I was doing was putting my teaspoon of peroxide into cold Postum without cream or sugar in it. I've cut out all sugar. I would have a piece of sharp cheddar cheese. I would take a bite before I swallow the peroxide/Postum solution, and take a couple of quick swallows and not breathe through my nose - just my mouth - then, I would take another bite of the sharp cheese to kill the peroxide taste. I would take a teaspoon, to 8 or 10 ounces of Postum. Some people even drink it with their meals. Some people recommend you take it an hour before eating in the morning, so that your stomach is real empty. I wouldn't be able to do that. I'm sure I would toss my cookies. I always waited an hour after eating. I found that if you had a little bit of food left in your stomach, that hadn't gone to your intestine yet, that that was best. The food remaining in your stomach was a little bit of a buffer for the peroxide."

Did you say you took ozone treatments twice? "That's right. They ozonate your blood. That, again, is just putting oxygen into your blood." Note: It is more complex than that, see section on ozone.

Where did you have that done? "At Gary Young's clinic. (Mexico) I think it's near Mesa. The headquarters are in Chula Vista, California. Dr. Donsbach has a clinic in the Baja Peninsula."

CORRESPONDENCE

HIGH BLOOD PRESSURE

Hugh Schoephoerster, Ph.D.   Anoka, Minnesota

"I started taking H_2O_2 5 years ago, blood pressure was 160/100, on hypertensive medicines... Now, it's 130/80, and no medicines. Started with minimal dosages of food grade to see what kind of relief resulted."

PERSISTANT VIRUS - BACK PAIN

Prof. Walter Fremanis   Oswego, NY

"Was ill for about a year with a virus that left me very weak feeling, similar to the Epstein-Barr virus, or "Yuppie" virus as reported in the news. Did not feel like doing anything, felt guilty about it as well, but the harder I tried to get out of this by taking vitamins, etc., the more tenacious it became. I was making the rounds of doctors and specialists who could find nothing wrong with me, but gave me lots of antibiotics, which did not seem to help, as there are no drugs that will kill a virus. One doctor said "either the virus will eventually die, or you will.""

"I sent for, and heard, Walter Grotz's tape. As soon as I took hydrogen peroxide, I could feel it go through my system. After starting the program, I did not have a flu or virus for about a year after that. I am presently on a maintenance program, and feel a great deal better."

"My wife, started it the same time as I. She had been in an accident, and displaced three discs. She's still affected by her injured discs, because the peroxide can't repair such a bad injury. Part of her pain was getting worse, and seemed to be arthritis settling into the injury site. She found great relief for her back pain with hydrogen peroxide!"

DEGENERATIVE JOINT DISEASE - COMMON COLD - HAIR LOSS

Mr. & Mrs. F.   Manlius, NY

"I Watched helplessly, as my wife, 62, became increasingly incapacitated by arthritis-like symptoms. We got a hopeless prognosis. Cortisone shots were recommended. We rejected the shots, and took aspirin. Getting out of a chair was a painful experience for her, as was her negotiating stairs. The use of her hands was becoming increasingly restricted. She frequently needed assistance, due to severe back pain, when straightening up after retrieving something from the floor. Normal household duties were becoming duties to be suffered through."

"We read about hydrogen peroxide in an obscure publication, sent for the information, and we both started on it. In spite of the fact that neither of us could stand to take the full suggested doses - within three weeks, my wife's condition had improved noticeably. Last week we spent part of the afternoon hunting woodchucks on a friend's farm. This entailed traversing some rough terrain and was something she has not been able to do for years."

"Three days after starting peroxide, a long-standing cold had vanished. As a closing comment, let me state that my wife, my two sons, and myself, have noticed a greatly reduced hair loss since starting on the peroxide treatments."

BACK AND SHOULDERS

G.R.   Oswego, NY

"I had difficulty with my back and shoulders. I could actually feel the H_2O_2 working it's way down from my head, down my neck, and into my back. I could feel different spots on body getting warmer whenever the H_2O_2 was working. The whole area loosened up. It's Great Stuff!"

ALLERGIES

A.R.   Oswego, NY

"While taking the hydrogen peroxide, I seemed to have less trouble with dust and sneezing, and also I seemed to breathe easier. I was having a reaction to our cats also, before the H_2O_2, when I'd pet them, I would sneeze, and my eyes would get watery and itch a lot. While taking the H_2O_2 it didn't happen."

INTERESTING OXYGENATION ITEMS

INTERFERON STIMULATES H_2O_2 PRODUCTION

Interferon may be an elaborate way to get H_2O_2 into the system. "Much of interferon's effectiveness is apparently due to the fact that it stimulates production of H_2O_2 and other oxygen intermediates... which are a key factor in reactivating the immune system."
- Journal of Interferon Research Vol 3, #2 1983 p. 143-151.

AGRICULTURE

"Farmers are regularly injecting 35% Food Grade H_2O_2 into their water supplies as a disinfectant at the rate of 8 ounces to each 1000 gallons of water or 10 to 30 parts per million. The Merck Index indicates it is used for this purpose."

"These farmers have noticed an increase in the milk production of their cows and also that the butterfat content goes up. Some farmers claim they have increased egg production and a drop in mortality rate. Some have said there is less feed consumption, while at the same time there is an increase in the weight of the bird. "The Diseases of Birds" by Robert Stroud, is a good book on bird diseases and peroxide. One farmer reported this was the first year his animals did not have coughing spells. Aqua Dynamics sells automatic liquid injectors that put the solution of your choice into water lines. Aqua Dynamics, 981-OT River Road, Reading, PA 19601"

"Others foliage sprayed their alfalfa and said it grew 6 inches taller at harvest time. They put 1 pint of 35% into 20 gallons of water per acre. They also reported it must be done before 7 A.M.
- ECHO NEWSLETTER Vol 2, #1

NEWS NOT HEARD YET

Why has there been no major media mention of these things? Why haven't we heard more about hydrogen peroxide, ozone, and the oxygen enhancing supplements, on the news? The news media ignored the Wright brother's first airplane flight, too, and for five years, did not attend any demonstration flights, despite constant invitations to do so. Perhaps nothing's changed. The big wheels turn slowly.

HYDROGEN PEROXIDE'S BAD PRESS

LIVING IN THE DUALITY

Nature's constant seeking of equilibrium is beautifully illustrated in the phenomenon where someone states an opinion or fact, and immediately there appears on the scene someone with the opposite opinion or fact. The use of hydrogen peroxide, ozone products, and other oxygenating products have already come under fire.

All of the bad press I have seen is only a lack of viewing a larger picture. I'll give you an example. If someone's skin came in contact with a powerful acid, like hydrochloric, and a severe burn resulted, some might speak out against hydrochloric acid. Yet, those same people have probably forgotten their bellies are full of it.

While we're on the subject of stomach acid, some researchers are discovering that the reduction of stomach hydrochloric acid production due to the aging process actually is a cause of incomplete digestion, and further accelerates aging. For this reason, many people now take time release HCL, stomach acid, supplements with their meals.

H_2O_2 CAUSING CANCER AND AGING?

Some sales literature for a competing oxygenation product claims "hydrogen peroxide is now proven harmful", and salesmen claim "it causes cancer and premature aging". Their relativistic viewpoint is true, it is a powerful oxidizer... used incorrectly, it could be dangerous, like in our stomach acid example. When you see these claims, remember, it is not against the law to publish fraudulent research studies. These articles are appearing in "health" magazines who run huge ads for the same salesmen, who also write the articles.

One spokesperson for this viewpoint, to prove it, even took straight undiluted 35% hydrogen peroxide and put it on yogurt cultures, killing them! Of course it did - putting that strong a concentration on any living thing would harm it!

I see the existence of this opposite viewpoint as a good thing, because a controversy will spur public debate, individual self responsibility, and more research. The last thing our society needs is people not taking the time to learn all about oxygenators, and either condemning them, or abusing them through overuse. Keep in mind, that these potent oxidizers all have a demonstrated, "window of effectiveness." Too small a dosage... nothing happens, too large a dosage... and you start killing cells. Between these two points is the range that works for each individual - the, "window." This concept will come up repeatedly in this book.

H_2O_2 KILLS FRIENDLY BACTERIA?

Another criticism, is that hydrogen peroxide "kills friendly bacteria in the intestines." Most friendly bacteria reside in the large intestine, approximately 20 feet distal to the duodenum where most of the H_2O_2 occurs. It is absorbed before it gets to the friendly bacteria. "Taking Aerox or hydrogen peroxide orally does not mean your long intestine is going to be invaded by the oxidizing activity. The active (unstable) hydrogen peroxide will most likely be used up in the stomach and most of it catalyzed into useful blood oxygen by the enzyme catalase long before it could get past the duodenum and into the intestine. The same goes for Aerox. You would need to take an overdose of both oxygenators to get activity into the intestines where your lactobacillus acidophilus are colonized." - Search For Health

FRIENDLY BACTERIA PRODUCE H_2O_2

"Incidentally, one of the "products" of active acidophilus (when they are functioning in your intestine) is hydrogen peroxide - the bacteria use this, as a means to control their natural enemy; candida albicans."
- Oxidation expert, Tom Valentine - Search For Health, Vol 1, #3

Let's not forget that the lymphocytes in your own blood also produce hydrogen peroxide all the time to fight disease. The point is, that, if hindered in their ability to do this, some means of restoring that ability is needed.

AMERICAN BIOLOGICS

Always in the market for a balanced viewpoint, I called one of the main disseminators of hydrogen peroxide bashing material, American Biologics (AB), 1180-OT Walnut Ave. Chula Vista, CA 92011, in mid July 1988.

They sell, to professionals only, a competing product called Dioxychlor (r), a U.S. legal homeopathic remedy containing minute amounts of chlorine dioxide, and operate a hospital in Tijuana. Their hospital clinic uses a number of therapies: Live Cell Therapy, where embryonic, fetal, calf cells are injected into the patient, laetrile, hydrazine sulfate, and others. Note: See the Stabilized Saline Oxygen - section for a further discussion on chlorine dioxide.

PEOPLE HURT?

I called them, as I had heard through my investigations of other sources, that AB allegedly claimed Dr. Donsbach and Dr. Farr had <u>allegedly</u> hurt people with their treatments, and these people had purportedly come to American Biologics Hospital for "repair" treatments afterwards.

On the phone they said - (quoting from a paper by the hospital's director, Robert Bradford [D.Sc.]) - *excessive* use of H_2O_2 is linked to: "Shutting down the immune system, producing clotting, irritation of the veins, rectal bleeding, shuts down the endocrine system, inhibition of the enzyme system, cellular damage, genetic damage, and enhancement of the aging process."

They claimed his conclusions were based upon, "empirical evidence, and 59 scientific papers." I repeatedly asked them how many people they have treated who were <u>actually hurt</u> by Dr. Donsbach, or Dr. Farr, and they were unable to give me even an approximate number that they based these conclusions on.

I further asked, "How could it be that all the people I interviewed (some in their 70's and taking H_2O_2 for over 7 years) had escaped all these <u>alleged</u> toxic side effects?" They suggested that: "They must have had exceptionally good immune systems." Then the question is, why were they sick? Remember, H_2O_2 has been reported as the first line of defense in our immune systems.

I was also told, that Dr. Farr was, "not now so much in favor of it as he was, and has, sort of, retracted some of his statements." And "even a low dosage was far beyond the safety range."

I Called Dr. Farr for verification of his so called, position reversal, and he said, in a word; "Fabrication." Dr. Farr is a research chemist, he has no products to sell. Far from retracting any earlier statements, he gives 10-15 treatments a day, and is giving international lectures in: Germany, England, and The Netherlands, to physicians, on methods of I.V. H_2O_2 use.

I asked Dr. Farr, "Where did these occasional inaccurate rumors come from?" Originally, he and Dr. Donsbach had encountered some phlebitis and vasculitis, but they quickly found out that their concentrations had far exceeded the therapeutic effectiveness. When Dr. Farr reduced the concentrations, the problems, to his knowledge, completely disappeared. He has had no further problems whatsoever.

I also asked Walter Grotz about this bad press with cited references, and he pointed out that "Nothing is 100%." He gave this example, to show us how scientists never all agree: during our first atomic test, a percentage of scientists said the atom bomb would never work. Another percentage said that if it did work, it would never stop reacting, continuing on, and consuming everything. These were the top scientists in the world.

So, when we stack up Walter Grotz's 6,000 medical references, all referring to some beneficial use of hydrogen peroxide, against around 59 research papers saying, "bad", then the weight of evidence is clearly on the side of "good".

H_2O_2 NEGATIVE REFERENCES

American Biologics sold me references in support of how harmful H_2O_2 was. The paper is very technical, and not easy for the average person to follow. The 57 page paper was entitled: "HYDROGEN PEROXIDE - THE MISUNDERSTOOD OXIDANT - by Bradford, Allen, and Culberet, 1987.

In it, we learn in one of the cited studies (Clinical research 15, p74 (1967), Fuson, R. L. et al.), the subject researchers apparently <u>denied</u> <u>8</u> <u>pigs 20%</u> <u>of</u> <u>their</u> <u>normal</u> <u>breathing (oxygen)</u> <u>requirements,</u> <u>put</u> <u>3%</u> H_2O_2 <u>(mixed with saline)</u> <u>directly</u> <u>into</u> <u>their</u> <u>hearts,</u> <u>and</u> <u>watched 5 of them</u> <u>die</u>. I'm surprised the other three lived. These animal studies serve as strong warnings indicating what can happen if you subscribe to the erroneous theory that "more is better" when dealing with potent oxidizers! A lay person slugging down peroxide could be his own worst enemy, if he doesn't use common sense. Note: See related section on SOD.

Please forgive me, if it seems I have strayed from objectivity in showing you all this, but how many people are going to be unnecessarily frightened away from the oxygenation subject, if I fail to show what lengths the opposition is going to?

Most of the references they sold me, did not state the concentrations used, and simply noted just the harm done to cells, chemicals, and processes from H_2O_2. What about the concentration levels? There is also a big debate going on about whether out of the body chemical reactions are the same as those in the body, because there are so many other agents and factors involved, and available to a living organism. Some concentrations listed in these references were above what Dr. Farr advocates as safe. Again, what about our safe levels, the "window of effectiveness" concept? American Biologics, itself, sells Dioxychlor(r), a compound generally regarded as safe, when administered in parts-per-million, and poison otherwise. It's a weak solution of chlorine dioxide. What would their research have shown, if high concentrations of poisonous chlorine dioxide was used, instead of H_2O_2?

ABH literature states that Dioxychlor (r) releases atomic oxygen. So does hydrogen peroxide, and many of the other competing oxygenators listed in this book. When Culbert and Bradford say (in the July 88 issue of "Health World" magazine) that Hydrogen Peroxide is an "activator and inducer" of Epstein-Barr Virus, and use as their proof an article written by their own organization, one wonders.

To say that sincere professionals are guilty of "intellectual perversion" (Actual quote from the ABH literature), simply because they have come up with differing viewpoints, is a waste of everyone's time, and draws the public attention away from all the exciting possibilities of fine tuning the various oxygenation processes being discovered and used.

On another front, while researching this book, I heard someone say "Hydrogen peroxide breaks up cell DNA", it's apparently the newest one liner. When I asked him for proof, or what he had to say about all the people claiming to have treated themselves without mishap, he recanted, and say he didn't really know if it did or not. The whole issue seems to be that most of this negativity is based upon theory, not actual case studies. The place where this type theorizing came from, was probably some study done outside of the human body. Remember that the basic premise is that whenever you have lipid peroxidation, you're going to have cell, RNA, and DNA breakdown. They're right, but it's not a bad thing. This is exactly how the peroxide seems to work. Introduced into a toxic (sick) body, it peroxidizes diseased cells and their DNA, along with harmful free radicals. It creates other free radicals to destroy them. In a following section of this book, Dr. Gerard Sunnen states that higher organisms have enzymes that repair RNA and DNA, and bacteria and viruses don't. That's why only the lower lifeforms die from these therapies, and the human cells are unaffected.

What the detractors might not be aware of, is Professor Halliwell's work: "Oxygen Radicals - A Common Sense Look At Their Nature And Medical Importance". In it, he proves that hydrogen peroxide is natural in the body. " Singlet O_2 is an especially reactive form of oxygen, capable of oxidizing many molecules, including membrane lipids. It's formation in O_2 (minus) generating systems has often been proposed, but clear cut evidence for a damaging role of singlet oxygen in such systems has not been obtained." Please note he said, "Not been obtained." Further, "There are a number of oxidation enzymes that produce H_2O_2 directly, examples being glycoly oxidation amino acid oxidases. SOD enzymes remove O_2- by dismutation reaction. So, if we accept that O_2- is formed *in vivo* in humans, then we must accept that H_2O_2 is produced as well. Indeed, H_2O_2 vapor is in expired human breath, a likely source is alveolar macrophages... That H_2O_2 is formed in vivo in humans is further supported by the presence of enzymes specific for it's removal: catalase, and glutathione peroxidase." - Professor B. Halliwell, Department of Biochemistry, University of London, King's College. Medical Biology, 1984, 62, 71-77.

I'll state again, that the two main questions are always: "Was the study done in a living body?" and, "What was the strength of the dosage?"

If we approach the health problem as one of an impaired immune function, and then use oxygenators, etc. (to bring the immune system back up to whatever 100% is, for each particular individual), then all we are doing is returning a patient to normal. Levels far above normal may indeed do harm.

DR. FARR STATES HIS H_2O_2 CONCENTRATIONS

Dr. Farr stated that in his intravenous injection work with H_2O_2, he used "0.0375 as an upper limit of concentration. From there, on down to 100 times weaker, is an effective range. And that's probably still 100 times greater than is necessary to completely stimulate your oxidative enzyme systems." I asked him if H_2O_2 has "shut down" anyone's immune system, as claimed by some detractors? He replied, "That won't happen, and I have the documentation to back it up." Early intravenous research used too strong concentrations, and had some problems (only at first) with vasculitis, but the H_2O_2 was, at that time, being mixed with other substances as well. He still cautioned, "With oral usage, some people quickly develop an irritated stomach."

The way a lot of this "rhubarb" got started, was back when new companies wanted to get aseptic H_2O_2 packaging. There were some articles brought up by their competition that the FDA had to deal with. In 1980, Japanese researchers had published a report that suggested hydrogen peroxide might induce gastritis and duodednal cancer in animals. Were they observing our "window of effectiveness" approach, or burning and mutating cells with too strong concentrations? And, what about species specificity? Many maintain that things like duodenal cancer in mice, may be solely because they are not human. (Assuming a correct dosage was used.)

Dr. Farr states he doesn't know how the body chemically handles H_2O_2 in the stomach, so he stays away from it, and goes the intravenous route. He states, the body may handle it OK, he just doesn't know about it. In any event, the FDA first investigated, and then discounted, the Japanese negative research that some were quoting. They ruled that: "there is insufficient evidence, from the Japanese Hiroshima study, and elsewhere, to conclude that hydrogen peroxide is a duodenal carcinogen." - Fed. Register.

DATA SHOWS NO TOXICITY

"We have lots of data now, showing that there is absolutely no toxicity, when used intravenously, that we can document at all. We've given 2,500 to 3,000 intravenous treatments now, (over the past three years) and no signs of toxicity, except irritations to the veins that occurred early in the study... At the concentrations we now use, buffering or pre-infusing with Heparin is not necessary. It was not an inflammatory condition, but a cytolytic. (Note: Cytolytic means cell lysis, or decomposition) This was entirely dependent upon the concentrations. Therefore, where you reduce your concentration, where it does not exceed roughly ten micro moles at the cell wall, you get away from the cytotoxic (cell burning) effect." - Dr. Farr.

CLYMER CLINIC - DR. HUGO VEITZ

As an example; I spoke with one of the 100 US doctors doing IV H_2O_2 treatments. Dr. Hugo Veitz, MD (IBOM member) who is with Clymer Health Clinic in Quakertown, PA. He gave ozone treatments for years, then the FDA decided to not allow ozone treatments. The FDA only heard from people using the wrong kind, or too much, ozone in their experiments. At the same time, they were unaware of medical ozone's widespread and excellent 30 year track record in Europe. As a result, Dr. Veitz, and many other doctors, had to switch to IV H_2O_2. He has treated over 60 people with repeated treatments, and hasn't had a single problem. He follows Dr. Farr's protocols, infusing slowly (about 1 1/2 to 2 hours for each treatment), with no buffering solutions, except saline or dextrose, and at low concentrations. He has tried .15% on himself, and has not had any problems either, except that he feels better and has a lot more energy.

There was one political problem Dr. Veitz ran into. One lady took 6 IV H_2O_2 treatments, and then, complained to the FDA that he was charging $60 per treatment, and it didn't do any good. She wasn't harmed in any way. He had told her from the start, that in most instances, a minimum of 10 treatments was needed. This is what experience has taught him to be the length of time necessary to achieve positive effects. She dropped out early.

Note: In the section on Dr. Koch, toward the end of this book, we see how; Self responsibility, diet, bowel condition, and repeated exposure to external disease causing conditions, contributes or detracts to the success of many of these therapies.

Many people, unable to find time to give their children love, send them to psychiatrists, hoping to have them "fixed", as if they were sending a car to the shop. Real health is not instant. I spoke to many doctors, before doing this book, and they all expressed the same sentiment: "I'm tired of working on people who won't take responsibility for their own health!" Some things happen slowly, they take time. The IV H_2O_2 patient has to be able to stick with the program. Dr. Veitz is at the Clymer Health Clinic, RD#3-OT Quakertown, PA 18951

THE GERSON INSTITUTE/THERAPY CENTERS

"I see in Dr. Max Gerson one of the most eminent geniuses in medical history." - Dr. Albert Schweitzer

Charlotte Gerson has continued with the goals of her late husband, Max. Teaching; methods for healing and preventing disease - particularly the so called "incurable" diseases. She takes great pains to stress that, healing is a total approach. Although the Gerson Therapy Centers use ozone and hydrogen peroxide, it is only a part of the treatment. Diet, lifestyle, and emotional /mental health, all need to be in balance.

The Gerson institute states that it can supply complete medical documentation for hundreds of people who once had "incurable" diseases, and are now free of them, by using their methods. They sell books, reports, and operate clinics in Mexico. They can be reached by writing to: Gerson Institute, P.O.Box 430-OT, Bonita, CA, 92002

WE NATURALLY PRODUCE FREE RADICALS

FREE RADICAL "An atom, or group of atoms, having at least one unpaired electron."   - American Heritage Dictionary

"If excess free radical activity occurs in our bodies, we end up with having more cells destroyed than we can create. With cell death, we have tissue death: with tissue death, we have organ death: with organ death, we have body death. It all begins at the cellular level with free radicals."

- Zane Baranowski, popular writer

"These things are so hard to document, most of them are someone's idea, because these chemical complexes, particularly free radicals, they exist for only fractions of a second. It's almost impossible to really understand what's happening or to document what's happening, because we don't have any good way of measuring. It's over so quick.. It happens before you know it."

"I.V. hydrogen peroxide inhibits free radical production in certain amounts because it oxidizes the iron. That's what makes it confusing, because it is a precursor of hydroxyl radicals, that's true. But only under certain conditions, and fortunately, those conditions apparently don't exist most of the time."
                                                          - Dr. Charles H. Farr

HYDROGEN PEROXIDE AND THE HYDROXYL RADICAL

There is a great debate over free radicals going on, one side says; "stop them" and the other side says, "Put the opposite ones together". Many studies claim that hydrogen peroxide causes cellular damage, because it is found in the body. These studies leave out the facts that "Hydrogen peroxide is necessary for membrane stability, an intermediate in oxidative respiration, a secondary messenger, necessary in thyroid metabolism, estrogen production, used by NK and PMN cells to destroy phagocytized organisms or immunocomplex material, and has been found to participate in many other metabolic functions...perhaps it's role in free radical damage has been misinterpreted. Although diatomic oxygen (paired free radicals) is reduced to superoxide by the addition of one electron, this reaction has not been isolated or quantitated in (in the body) studies."
                                                          - IBOM Newsletter

FREE RADICALS

Probably the best known thing about free radicals is that they are blamed for diseases in an early "James Bond-007" spy movie. Remember, it's now an old movie. Since then, we have found out a lot more about them. Because of their makeup, free radicals react with other substances quickly, and have very short lives, less than a second. Like people; some assist balance, and some detract. We all know that breathing automobile exhaust can kill us. The reason is that carbon monoxide (CO) is taken up by the blood more quickly than oxygen - so, we would suffocate. This carbon monoxide is a free radical. The way our bodies decrease the carbon monoxide in our blood is by adding to it another free radical, our friend, oxygen (O1). Together, they balance each other out and we exhale the result - carbon dioxide (CO2) (making plants very happy). They are not "bad" as once thought, but necessary for balance.

Walter Grotz on Free Radicals:

"Show me one. I've never seen one. These are all just theories."

BODILY PRODUCTION OF H_2O_2

Our bodies produce free radicals to attack invading organisms. Leukocytes (white cells in the blood) produce a natural hydrogen peroxide. They do this from a specialized part of themselves that functions like an organ, (an "organelle") called a peroxisome. They send out a layer of hydrogen peroxide which surrounds and destroys harmful microbes. The hydrogen peroxide breaks down into water and oxygen (O_1). This form of oxygen (O_1)

is a free radical. Therefore, it is unstable. It attaches to the most unstable structure around it; a virus or harmful microbe fits the bill. It disrupts them electrically, and this kills the bacteria - or disrupts the virus - and the white cells digest the remains. Any leftover peroxide is neutralized by catalase, an enzyme also produced by the peroxisome. The cycle of defense is completed. This is our immune system at work.

SOME SUGGESTED FUTURE PROTOCOLS

Although we have witnessed some amazing results, we are really only at the beginning of completely understanding these wonderful applications of hydrogen peroxide. My personal opinion is that we should promote individually determined limits on it's use, otherwise, the general population will incorrectly think "more is better" and possibly do themselves harm. Here are some possible suggestions (not prescriptions) that future health care professionals may want to incorporate:

1) Anyone with a serious illness should only take it according to the advice of qualified health care professionals, or experts who are familiar with it's use, so together you can monitor the healing process.

2) Anyone who doesn't have a serious illness, and is just taking it as a cleanser or preventative, might consider using it sparingly, or if continually, for no more than about a month at a time, and not in high concentrations. After someone takes hydrogen peroxide, they might consider ingesting acidophilus cultures, either in pills or live culture yogurt, which help regenerate the friendly intestinal digestive flora, in case any were destroyed. If you don't have AIDS or cancer or the like, there is no need to totally saturate yourself with too much hydrogen peroxide. You might risk unbalancing your system.

3) Anyone who takes hydrogen peroxide, for any reason, might consider also taking a SOD (super oxide dismutase) antioxidant enzyme complex, which is specially made from wheat sprouts. It's mentioned in the last section of this book. In case any excess, or harmful, free radicals were formed by the hydrogen peroxide, then they will probably be neutralized by the antioxidants. It would probably be best to take them separately.

4) Although hydrogen peroxide starts out slightly pH acidic, it can create an alkaline pH in the body. This would be due to a system compensating rebound effect, similar to lemon juice, especially if used by non-meat eaters. If you introduce vitamin C, an acid, into this environment, you might get a very uncomfortable "bubbling" inside your body. The acid could disassociate some hydrogen away (creating excess hydrogen), which creates a situation of excess alkalinity. This allows an undesirable pH reaction which acts the same as if you were to combine two opposites - an acid and an alkali (base) - in the lab. Note: I did this once, while mistaking a cleansing reaction for an illness. I thought I was going to "pop" from internal bubbling, after I took vitamin C.

SUGGESTED DOSAGES

For a current list of Food Grade 35% suppliers, contact ECHO. For the current suggested dosage levels and protocols, contact ECHO and IBOM. Addresses listed in the back of this book. Also see the last part of this book for other ways people are getting peroxide into their bodies.

STRESSED IMMUNE SYSTEMS

If diet, pollution, lifestyle, etc., have weakened our immune systems enough, then the immune response process doesn't happen as it should. The body is an amazing piece of work, and is also just like a machine. If given good fuel (natural food), clean lubrication (natural oils), aspirated correctly (proper breathing and clean air), and operated properly (in harmony), it will last a long time. What differentiates us from a machine, is twofold: *Our ability to love, and, to be creative!* A way to love yourself, and make good use of your creativity, would be to find ways of changing your lifestyle to get more oxygen into your body.

ANTIOXIDANTS AND CANCER

"It becomes clear that two factors are associated with carcinogenesis: one is absence (or a very low concentration) of intracellular oxygen, and the other is a high concentration of certain antioxidants. The nature of these antioxidants (AO'S) is not known, but the most likely candidates are the synthetic substances present in processed food products... Such a condition gives rise to a situation, in which no lipid peroxidation products are formed, and thus no powerful cell division inhibitors are available."
- Rationale For Treatment of Cancer with Ozone, B. Lipinski, Ph.D.

AEROBIC VS. ANAEROBIC (OR) OXIDATION VS. FERMENTATION.

ANSWER IS RIGHT UNDER THEIR NOSES

A nurse who works in medical research said to me,"It's so simple. I don't know why I never thought of it. When we're working with cell cultures in the lab, if we want the cells to mutate, we turn down the oxygen. To stop them, we turn the oxygen back up."

"Cancer, above all other diseases, has countless secondary causes. but there is ONLY ONE PRIME CAUSE. SUMMARY: THE PRIME CAUSE OF CANCER IS THE REPLACEMENT OF THE NORMAL OXYGEN RESPIRATION OF BODY CELLS BY AN ANAEROBIC CELL RESPIRATION."
- Otto Warburg, twice Nobel Laureate

"Lack of cellular oxygen supply is probably the most common cause of cell injury and may also be the ultimate mechanism of damage."
- Robbins and Cotran (W.B. Saunders) Pathologic Basis of Disease

"Since Warburg's discovery, this difference in respiration has remained the most fundamental (and some say, only) physiological difference consistently found between normal and cancer cells. Using cell culture studies, I decided to examine the differential responses of normal and cancer cells to *changes in the oxygen environment*. The results that I found were rather remarkable. I found that "normal" O2 tension actually maximized the growth of the cancer tissue, and that *high O2 tensions were lethal to cancer tissue*, 95% being very toxic, whereas in general, normal tissues were not harmed by high oxygen tensions. Indeed, some normal tissues were found to require high O2 tensions....It does seem to demonstrate the possibility that if the O2 tension in cancer tissues can be elevated, then the cancer tissue may be able to be killed selectively, as it seems that the cancer cells are incapable of handling the O2 in a high O2 environment."
- J.B. Kizer: Biochemist/Physicist, Gungnir Research, Portsmith, OH

Hydrogen peroxide is not only important to the body's normal function, but it's oxidizing ability can be used to: oxidize weak old white blood cells, destroy immunocomplexes, kill bacteria, protozoa, and yeast, inhibit viruses, oxidize fatty deposits on the arterial walls, increase oxygen tension between cells, stimulate oxidative enzymes, return elasticity to the arterial walls, dilate coronary vessels, and regulate membrane transport.
                    - From the IBOM Newsletter, Vol 1, No.2 April 1987

HYDROGEN AND OXYGEN
- NECESSARY ADVERSARIES IN THE BODY

Hydrogen, by itself, is a colorless, highly flammable gas. It is the most abundant element in the universe, and the lightest of all gasses.

Oxygen is a colorless, odorless gas, that comprises about 45.6% of the earth's crust, and, at present, 20.95% of our atmosphere. It combines with most elements, and is required for respiration, and most combustion.

Hydrogen (H) and Oxygen (O) are two gasses necessary for life. Combined with carbon and nitrogen, they form proteins. Combined with carbon, they form carbohydrates. Combined with each other, they make water, and if you saturate water with extra oxygen, you get hydrogen peroxide (H_2O_2). Oxygen, along with other gasses, is the breath of life. All these elements and compounds exist in our blood. The creation and dissolution, or "yin and yang", of existence, is exemplified by hydrogen and oxygen.

HYDROGEN

Hydrogen is associated with the properties of: solidification, integration, and concentration. It brings together a matrix of energies, evolving these energies into solid forms. If the hydrogen characteristic properties are allowed to continue on unchecked, then the form gets denser and denser. Finally, extreme hardness settles in. These properties are the ones that bring the form of our bodies into existence, out of the DNA. It builds cells, and if left unmodulated, makes them hard and brittle. These effects are balanced by the action of oxygen.

OXYGEN

Oxygen is associated with: dissolving, disintegrating, and deconcentrating. Oxygen represents the opposite pole of creation, being the fluid substance that hydrogen builds life forms from, at the beginning, and after they have lived their useful life, erasing the created forms back to a fluid state. Oxygen keeps cells clean and flexible, and removes unneeded structure.

Generally speaking, in our bodies, hydrogen makes things hard, oxygen softens them up. Remember this, as it is a key to our subjects.

EXAMPLES

Examples of these two actions are: the industrial food processors using hydrogen to thicken vegetable oil into margarine, and nature using the rapid oxidation process of fire to decompose something quickly. In our bodies, they perform similar functions, the hydrogen gives our bodies structure, and the oxygen burns the food that is used to make the structure, as well as cleaning up afterwards.

HOW HYDROGEN AND OXYGEN AFFECT HEALTH

A clean body is more flexible. If there is not enough oxygen, then both the solidifying function, and incomplete combustion, occur to excess. Leftover incomplete combustion byproducts collect in our cells. We say that the body is toxic, or has a buildup of waste products. Under these conditions, the immune system has a hard time fighting off disease. All the cells and fluids have become "dirty". In other words, if our body's oxygen level drops too low, then we don't have much energy. If a chronic low oxygen condition is allowed to continue, we can't manufacture healthy cells, "burn" energy, or remove the "ashes". Under this increasing stress, the immune system tries harder and harder to do it's job, but is so overwhelmed from trying to clean out the "dirt" that illness might result. Note: See also, the section on the immune system.

CONSEQUENCES OF LOW OXYGEN

If our air supply (oxygen) is cut off, the waste products can't be burned at all. First there is brain damage, and, if continued long enough, we expire. Ever notice how, after exercise that makes you breathe heavily, you feel refreshed? If the body oxygen levels are maintained at proper levels, the feeling of well-being might be continual. Consider, also, that most older people are "brittle", when it comes to their body parts. They usually have built up waste products in their cells, don't get enough exercise, have eaten a lifetime of hydrogenated, oxygen deficient foods, and are "short breathers". They are not getting enough oxygen, and the solidifying characteristics of hydrogen are dominating.

HOW WE ARRIVE AT A LOW OXYGEN LEVEL

Body oxygen levels can drop for a variety of reasons, the obvious ones are injury or disease. Air should have about 20% oxygen, but, in the cities, it can drop to 10%. Ancient air bubbles, that were trapped in amber, have been analyzed as containing twice as much oxygen as we now have in our air. Tap water loses oxygen from chlorine, and from not being aerated. Cooking drives the extra oxygen out of vegetables. Have you noticed how many raw juice and vegetable health diets have been proposed over the years? Antibiotics kill friendly bacteria that produce H_2O_2 in the body. Processed and hydrogenated foods cause the circulatory system to spend more time hauling out toxins than carrying in oxygen.

HOW MUCH DO WE BREATHE DAILY?

"In a 24 hour day, the adult man uses... (approx.) 8 pounds of oxygen..." - A. Schatz, discoverer of streptomycin, in Cancer News Journal, v.12, n.2, p.6, June 1977.

The average man consumes 6 to 8 pounds of oxygen, 4 pounds of food, and 2 pounds of water. More oxygen goes into our bodies than the other two combined. I would say oxygen is important.

JAPANESE SELL OXYGEN

Some ancient cultures installed big pipes on hilltops and pumped fresh mountain air down to the congested cities below.

First in Japan, and now in the U.S., they sell small bottles of oxygen complete with a little mask. Well-known Japanese department stores have even set up "oxygen bars", where customers can inhale scented oxygen. Canned oxygen, aimed at the sports market, has been sold to athletes in sporting goods stores as of a few years ago.

Tokyo's Takashimaya department store said they sold more than 300 gift sets of oxygen during the 1987 December season. Several stores offer gift sets of oxygen combined with sporting goods, health drinks or mineral water. A five quart canister of 95% concentrated oxygen, (weighing about six ounces) gives the impression that one is holding a can of nothing. But at $11 a can, you hope you've bought something. The can contains enough oxygen to last about two minutes, or 60 to 80 breaths.

The companies producing the canisters claim that they relieve post sports fatigue, and can be used to refresh yourself while working or driving. They admit, for a healthy person, the effects may be minimal.

ESSENTIAL FATTY ACIDS
- THEIR ROLE IN OXIDATION

According to the work of West German Physicist Dr. Johanna Budwig, Ph.D.: The red blood cells in the lungs give up carbon dioxide and take on oxygen. They are then transported to the cell site via the blood vessels, where, they release their oxygen into the plasma. This released oxygen is "attracted" to the cells by the "resonance" of the "pi-electron" oxidation-enhancing fatty acids. Otherwise, oxygen cannot work it's way into the cell. She published technical papers as far back as 1951 proving that "electron-rich fatty acids," play the decisive role in "respiratory enzymes, which are the basis of cell oxidation...". Might one of the respiratory enzymes she refers to be CoQ10? Or Superoxide Dismutase?

So, according to Dr. Budwig, we should eat these essential polyunsaturated fatty acids to enhance oxygenation. They can be found naturally in carotene, in saffron, and in flaxseed oil.

These electron-rich fats "resonate with the wavelength of the sun's light and control the entire scope of our bodies vital life functions!" says Dr. Budwig.

Conversely, according to Dr. Budwig, if we eat anything hydrogenated, it defeats the purpose of oxygenation. She gives the examples of margarine, which is oil with hydrogen bubbled through it to solidify it, or fried foods. Read the label of what you're about to eat, does it say "hydrogenated"? Is there an alternative?

THE BEST OIL?

Udo Erasmus, author of the modern classic: "Fats and Oils" was recently interviewed on the Radio Free America satellite talk show. He has traveled extensively to interview all the commercial oil producers. He is an expert on oils, and has stated the best oil for human consumption is fresh flaxseed oil prepared in the proper way. He cautions that some natural food companies took linseed oil destined for the paint market, "dead oil - no life left in it", and sold it to health food stores. His investigations have shown that presently, the only source of pure, fit for human consumption, flaxseed oil in the U.S. is the Spectrum Naturals brand, which is called "Veg-Omega-3 Certified Organic Flax Oil". Flaxseed oil is never to be heated, as this will destroy the benefits. It can be put on salads, or eaten by itself. Spectrum Naturals, 133-OT Copeland St. Petaluma, CA 94952.

Flaxseed oil was, at one time, a crop in the U.S., even being shipped overseas. Unfortunately, the FDA has ruled against a company trying to import it, saying that it is not a food, but a food "additive" because, "you put it on something, like a salad". It can be purchased in Canada and Europe.

AGING RELATED TO OXYGEN TRANSPORT

Oxidation is a process of delivering nutrients, digesting our food, and releasing energy. Oxygen cleans up after this process too. Oxygenation could theoretically slow the aging process by keeping our cells so clean, that they would only wear out very slowly. Instead of aging by toxins, we would only have to contend with the scientifically admitted effects of cosmic radiation. The famous legends of the "fountains of youth" may have been referring to very oxygenated water. - From Mike Brown, Mechanical engineer and oxygenation researcher.

In "The Nutrition and Dietary Consultant", we find: "Aging. When there is a lack of oxygen, the body is unable to assimilate Vitamin C properly. There is a collagen breakdown. A lack of oxygen is why body organs grow old, permitting arteries and veins to harden. It is the primary cause of strokes and degeneration of the brain." - Sonya C. Starr, B.S., N.C.

Note: Also refer to the sections on SOD for aging related topics.

ALCOHOLIC & DRUG CRAVINGS AND OXYGEN

We get "high" from drinking because alcohol robs the brain of oxygen. Alcohol and drug cravings are reduced significantly by oxygenation. In fact, I had a personal experience with the effects of H_2O_2 and alcohol.

I rarely ever drink alcohol since I wised up to it, and I've lost any cravings (I assume this was due to my self oxygenating experiences), but I have a drinking story to tell you. Once upon a time a few years back, after being on peroxide for about 6 months, I went to the Kentucky Derby. Unless you've been there, or lived in Kentucky, you don't know the enormity of the event.

Surrounded with good friends, and in the spirit of the occasion, I ended up drinking beer and Kentucky whiskey all day. I started noticing my friends getting looser and looser, and then downright intoxicated. I was very puzzled that I didn't feel anything, especially since I was keeping right up with them, "consuming mass quantities"! Only late in the day (that started at 7 am), did I get some of the artificial party feelings, but they remained slight.

Then a realization hit me, "Like a hot kiss at the end of a wet fist" (Firesign Theatre quote), I realized that I probably had such a high level of oxygen in my body, that the alcohol was immediately oxidized, and, what did get through, wasn't able to rob my brain of oxygen significantly. My friends finally crashed, and I was wide awake, and never got a hangover.

The only side effect I experienced was the next morning, when I did have an anal burning sensation, I assume this was probably from the cross-purpose chemical interaction.

86

ALCOHOL AND DRUG ADDICTION

Let's take addiction as an example. Ignore the psychological factors in our example, and assume they are not physically created through the glands. Now look at how our bodies are always seeking balance. The cravings of drug addiction have been anecdotally reported to be reduced by oxygenation methods. Any body craving is a signal that there is a condition of "too much of something" in the cells. The craving is for the intake of that something's opposite balancer(s).

We now hear from scientists that most alcoholics are genetically predisposed to having certain compounds in their bodies that make them crave alcohol. These compounds build up, ready to dissolve alcohol, and if there is no alcohol, then they force you to get some. Nicotine, drugs, the same addictive mechanisms can be created by continual overindulgence.

If the cells storing these substances "at the ready", ready to dissolve the drugs, are cleaned by oxygenation and returned to the childhood DNA state of cleanliness, if there is no more foreign substance in the body creating an imbalance, where will the cravings come from?

WEIGHT LOSS

There are estimated to be over 80 million overweight people in the U.S. today. In his book, "Juice Fasting" Dr. Paavo Airola states that obesity is our biggest killer, and overweight people are twice as likely to contract a disease. Besides breathing, we get oxygen from our food. Clean, healthy bodies utilize foods more efficiently and effectively than bodies full of waste. Many oxygenated people report that the need to eat is greatly diminished, since the food consumed is so thoroughly utilized. Food cravings have many origins, but one is the body, trying to get more oxygen to the cells. If we increase our oxygen levels over time, then the appetite might be reduced to more normal levels.

BODY TEMPERATURE & OXYGENATION RATES

To give you a perfect example of how central oxygenation is to life, feel your skin, now blow on your hands. Where do you think all that heat comes from? 98.6 degrees comes from oxidation! The warm air of our breath is mostly carbon dioxide, CO_2. We burn our food in our cells by combining carbon products with oxygen for a source of energy.

This is also the area where we might get into trouble. What if there's not exactly enough oxygen in our body? The body is wonderfully adaptive. It's prime directive is survival, so, it will attempt to burn food anyway, even without enough oxygen around to sustain the process. The result of this incomplete reaction is: carbon with only one oxygen atom attached instead of 2. This is CO, not CO_2. Carbon monoxide, CO, is an unnatural product. It's the main poison in car exhaust, and it's not readily eliminated from the body. It actually acts as a harmful free radical de-oxidizer! CO poisons our systems further by irritating our organs and cells, destroying hemoglobin in the blood, and combining with, and using

87

up, more of our body's beneficial free radical oxygen. People around car exhaust usually have low oxygen levels because of this.

SYMPTOMS ALLIED WITH LOW BODY TEMPERATURE

This incomplete combustion process also lowers our body temperature, and medicine now has classifications of people as having subnormal temperatures. Subnormal temperature "types" commonly have one or more of the following symptoms: headache, dizziness, insomnia, constipation, faint-feeling, loss of appetite, heart palpitations, bad kidneys, menstrual problems, cold hands and feet (and various other symptoms), all of which might be due to an oxygen impoverished blood supply.

OZONE HAS NORMALIZED BODY TEMPERATURES

People who have only fractionally "below normal" body temperatures may show the same or even greater symptoms than people a number of degrees low. It has been demonstrated that people given repeated ozone treatments, have had their body temperatures rise to normal, and problems disappear.

- Condensed from the IBOM Newsletter.

HBO - HYPERBARIC OXYGEN THERAPY

One of the most common questions I'm asked is: *"Why don't people just go into an oxygen chamber?* Sitting in a high-pressure oxygen chamber is also known as, OHP, Oxygen under high pressure, or HBO, Hyperbaric oxygen. It was first used medically in England, three centuries ago, to treat North Sea industrial divers with "the bends". It also works well in conditions where oxygenation has been reduced, and anaerobic infective bacteria are apt to flourish, as in gangrene. In Dr. Farr's talk we saw how he considers this method expensive and inefficient compared with hydrogen peroxide. Here are some historical references on the use of HBO.

GANGRENE

In 1965, the British Medical Journal printed a report stating "Hyperbaric oxygen has saved both life and limb... One of the most dramatic features is the almost immediate arrest of the disease (gangrene) and the improvement in the patient's condition. Hyperbaric treatment is combined with antibiotics, and surgery is deferred until after the treatment is complete, when the operation can often be confined to simple procedures such as the removal of necrotic sloughs (dead tissue) and skin grafting."

TOO LITTLE STIMULATED CANDIDA

Dr. Boguslav H. Fischer of the New York University School of Medicine wrote, in 1971, that "..when damaged tissue cannot utilize oxygen, it has no defense against infection." He also adds this interesting note about this oxygenation method - that, Candida and other infective organisms can be stimulated by oxygen if the pressure isn't sufficiently high.

Note: Please keep in mind this phenomenon, when you get to the
sections on hydrogen peroxide and ozone's reported "window" of
effectiveness.

USED ON BONE INFECTIONS

Many   U.S.   doctors have used   OHP (oxygen,   high pressure) on
chronic osteomyelitis (bone infection) with success. Many of these
also concluded that it is not the OHP that influences disease, but
that   it   stimulates   the   body's   immune   system   to   attack   it.
Scientists now think that both mechanisms are involved.

REPLACED TRANSFUSIONS

Dr. George B. Hart, on May 20th, 1974, published in the
Journal of the AMA that 3 Jehovah's Witnesses (who wouldn't
accept transfusions) were saved by OHP. "Treatment with hyperbaric
oxygen resulted in dramatic improvement, with reversal of the signs
and   symptoms of hypoxia (lack of oxygen) in all three patients".
Although   they had a limited amount of blood, it became oxygen
saturated.

CHRONIC VERTIGO

Chronic vertigo patients received benefits from OHP applied by
a Dr. Nair at Norwalk hospital in Connecticut, and the New England
Journal of medicine reported, in 1969, that senile patients
improved mentally with OHP.

OZONE

OZONE HUMOR

    "Air pollution (smog) is an Auto Immune disease."

              - From the Author of "Medical Dark Ages".

LAB RESEARCHER DISCOVERS OZONE HEALS

MERLIN

This section is presented to show that there is, quite possibly, a lot we don't know about establishing dosages, protocols, and types of "ozones". It is condensed from a series in the Journal of Borderland Research, Garberville, CA, Sept/Oct, 1986 by "Merlin" (penname). My efforts to find him have not been successful.

"MERLIN'S" PAPER TITLED "OZONE TOXICITY"

A research chemist (Merlin) was employed by a firm to evaluate an ozone machine they were considering using to delay fruit decay in agricultural warehouses. They had always heard that ozone was toxic, so they set out to find out about it.

SPECIAL OZONE GENERATOR

The chemist secured the machine produced by the "APSEE(?)" company. - Phonetic spelling. (Note: No further information is available as we go to press. If you know about this person or company, please write the author.) This ozone generator was unlike some others, in that it wasn't UV powered, but even at full power, there was no spark, only a blue-violet plasma glow. It funneled air over charged (5000v) stainless steel and special composite ceramic disc "sandwiches". It was supposed to impart extra electrons to the air going through, and these electrons would attach themselves to airborne microbes, spores and particulates. The electrons would impart a negative charge, and make them precipitate out of the air.

MOUSE EXPERIMENT

The chemist took a severely diseased laboratory mouse, and put it in the full stream of the output of the device. He assumed it was dying anyway, and he thought he would kill the mouse with the ozone, and then dissect it, to find out exactly why it died. The mouse had no fur on its head and neck, and was covered with open sores that it violently scratched. It's right eye was opaque with cataract, and it had a tumor on it's stomach that was so large, that it's feet could barely reach the ground.

OZONE DIDN'T KILL

He turned the machine on full. After some initial agitation, the mouse started building a nest. To the amazement of the chemist, instead of dying, within a few hours, the mouse stopped scratching. By the next morning all his inflamed sores had dried up, and scabbed over. The mouse received a total of sixty continuous hours of full-power treatment. He was placed in a normal cage for six weeks, to study any long term effects. Within a week; all sores were healed, the scabs were gone, and the skin became soft and normal-looking. At two weeks, the skin had it's color back, new fur was growing, and the tumor was smaller. By six weeks, the tumor was completely gone and the eye was pink, clear and responsive! From then on, he lived a long life, and sired many litters.

In this experiment, the ozone did not kill, but healed! There must be a lot of dynamics unaccounted for with ozone usage.

THE DIFFERENT OZONES

Clark E. Thorp, Chairman, Dept. of Chemistry and Chemical Engineering of the Armour Research Foundation of Illinois Institute of Technology, published some interesting observations in the Feb. 1950 edition of Medicine and Surgery, Vol. 19, No. 2. He showed that electrically produced ozone, produced from air, was highly toxic. But, ozone from pure oxygen wasn't. The main difference was that air produced ozone had a lot of nitrogen oxides present with it, and the pure oxygen ozone didn't. Another researcher was reported to have produced a less toxic air/ozone mixture by using low humidity air. This lack of humidity prevented a lot of arcing in the ozone generator's electrodes. Notice that the "Apsee" machine, used on the lab mouse, had no electrical arcing. It produced a cold plasma ozone.

HEAT AND WATER MAKE ACIDS IN OZONE

Nitrogen oxide (NOX) gases are formed when nitrogen and oxygen are combined under heat. Among these is $2NO_2$, nitrogen dioxide, a reddish brown gas that's deadly poison. When combined with water, as in air humidity, it forms NHO_3, NITRIC ACID! This means that proper levels of ozone aren't toxic, but the contaminants, thermally induced during it's manufacture, are!

HOT SPARK OZONE KILLED MOUSE

To test this, our intrepid chemist built a "hot spark" type generator, and it's output produced an amber colored gas, matching nitric acid. This was the opposite of the ozone from the earlier cold process unit, which was colorless. New test mice were placed within the hot spark/amber gas output. The gas was recirculated over and over, producing high concentrations. They expired in two to three minutes. In another test, more mice were placed in the output of the cold/clear gas, which was recirculated continually, to also produce a high concentration. They died in five minutes.

The differences: in the last two examples, there was too high a concentration used. There was severe internal bleeding in the hot spark/amber gas ozone subjected mice, probably because nitric acid was formed from the air, and also from contact with moist areas of the lung, which eroded the tissues. However, the mice subjected to too high concentrations of the cold/clear ozone died as well, but showed no bleeding. Upon dissection, Merlin did notice they all had edema (fluid swelling). He surmised that this abnormal swelling of the cells had caused their suffocation. He said that this was due to too much oxygen being released into the tissues at one time.

92

In looking at these various experiments, we can conclude that we've got two very different types of "ozone gasses" that most everyone incorrectly assumes are the same: one is not just ozone, and always very toxic, and the other is the contaminant free one, which is pure natural ozone, and only toxic at too high of a concentration.

OZONE NOT ALWAYS TOXIC

According to these experiments, broadly saying "Ozone is toxic", is an uninformed opinion, due to oversimplification. It's what you hear from the media, which usually only has time for "one-liners". Being highly oxidative, ozone combines readily with almost anything, and if contaminated, *the* **contaminants** are the toxins, not the ozone used at proper levels! Here's an example. The FDA says ozone irritates the mucosa of the lungs. What "type" of ozone are they referring to? Even if the correct type is used, consider what happens when someone breathes it. It starts to oxidize all the pollutants, tar, pot, microbes, etc. in the lung tissues, and the subjects begin coughing, as a means of naturally cleaning themselves out. Therefore, because of this coughing as a natural means of expelling oxidized toxins, the FDA says "ozone" is an irritant. All the ozone is doing, is to cause toxins to be decomposed and expelled. The toxins are the irritants. I've personally spoken with unharmed people who breathe pure natural ozone (at low levels) all the time. You breathe it yourself, on clear sunny days outdoors, and after lightning storms. Ozone is unfairly given a bum rap. It is Nature's natural disinfectant. It's the "fresh" smell on outdoor laundry. Did breathing that ever hurt you?

Note: We interrupt here, to interject, that Andrew Pincon, President of an ozone company reviewed later, states that: "Actually, if air is your input gas, all electronic methods of ozone manufacture produce some nitric acid, nitrous oxides, and other nitrogen compounds. The amount is much smaller without thermal bonding from sparking. Even negative ion generators produce ozone, and form minute amounts of nitric acid as well, and that's a cold plasma discharge, too. About 3% of your output will be various nitrogen by-products". Some maintain this is too small an amount to worry about, if used wisely. All the thousands of ion generators in use don't have any problems.

Please note: As I stated in the beginning of the book, none of this is meant to be therapeutic or healthcare advice for humans or animals. Do not assume it is. In the US it is illegal to do so under FDA rules. These and all other accounts given in this book are only reports of research and experiences. They are meant to spur public discussion of these overlooked subjects.

Merlin's tale continued in the next issue of BSRF, under "Electron Healing," Nov-Dec Journal of Borderland Research, 1986.

GENERATOR DESIGN

The subject cold plasma/ozone generator utilizes stacks of stainless steel and special dielectric ceramic discs of an unknown composition. Other generators use materials that may start out producing cold process ozone, but soon break down by erosion, and start sparking, producing the nitrogen dioxide acid contaminated ozone.

The subject process development chemist wrote that he observed effective treatment of the following conditions by the cold process ozone: Shingles (Herpes Zoster), Post herpetic neuralgia, Venereal Herpes, Skin Cancer, London Flu, Post surgical incisions, Third degree burns (pain & healing), Gangrene, Purulent staph infections, & Fungal Disease. Note: Again, I do not claim this as a cure.

MAN TREATS FUNGUS

He gives an example where a man suffered for 30+ years with an exotic fungal foot infection that would break out recurringly, leaving him unable to walk. Military and civilian medical care, including radiation, did nothing for it. His feet were placed in plastic trash bags, secured at the knees, and the cold process ozone fed into and through the bag, then exhausted outside. He had three cold process ozone treatments, of 25 minutes each, one every other day. Since then, he had no further outbreaks.

PLEASE NOTE: In any of the applications where the ozone air is used at these therapeutic levels, adequate forced ventilation of the treatment room is required. Strong concentrations of ozone are an irritant to the patient and operator's mucous membranes. Also, the power settings must be lower, as the gas will concentrate in the bag. I have talked with an ozone worker who has chronic infections from being near too much ozone, too often, leading to lung irritation over the years.

Note: This "plastic bagging" method is used by the Hansler group in Germany, and is a preferred method of treating severe burns, so nothing touches the burn site. They report that pain is greatly reduced, and rapid healing effected. It looks like burn victims might not have to suffer some of the agony once thought unavoidable. This should be tested, and developed here in the U.S.

RESEARCHER EXPERIMENTS ON SELF

Our researcher tried an experiment on himself. He accidentally severely burned himself with a hot welding rod. Leaving it untreated, it got very infected. It was swollen, draining, and throbbing, full of pus. He finally subjected his wound to a 30 minute direct exposure to the output of the machine. Upon arising the next morning, the towel he wrapped around the burn (for nightly drainage) was dry, the swelling subsided, and the large red inflammation had narrowed to a small strip. The wound had a dry scab over it which fell off 5 days later, without any permanent scarring. It was of particular interest to his physician that the infection was so rapidly (7.5 hours) assimilated into his system without any swelling of lymph nodes or secondary toxic reactions.

MERLIN'S OBSERVATIONS, AFTERTHOUGHTS AND THEORIES

We know that ozone works directly on bacteria, fungi, and viruses. This doesn't explain how application to the skin can resolve deep tissue problems. A possible explanation might be found in the 1971 work of Dr. Sutzkiyo Uozumi, Ph.D., a Japanese physicist.

JAPANESE PHYSICIST STUDIES OZONE

Dr. Uozumi revealed, through balanced mathematical and chemical equations, that airborne oxygen, when exposed to dense, high velocity electron plasma (without any heat from electrode sparking), will form into higher atomic groupings like O_{10}. This is through alterations in the individual atomic valences of the oxygen atom. Once this highly unstable "Super Oxygen" is released, it very quickly tries to return to the more stable O_2. In it's rapid decay from O_{10} down to O_9, O_8, O_7, O_6, O_5, O_4, O_3, and O_2, it randomly gives off electrons that encounter other previously unaffected oxygen molecules, and impacts them, giving them some of it's secondary free electrons. These oxygen molecules are transformed by this process into higher forms, from O_2 to O_3, to O_4+ etc., which in turn break down into O_5, O_4, O_3, etc., also releasing electrons and creating other higher forms, which then break down and give off electrons, etc.

CASCADING OZONE

This process is called, an "electron avalanche effect", or "secondary electron effect". This shows that oxygen does not need to go through the electron plasma, it only needs to come in contact with other higher oxygen forms. Another major point, is that this rapid giving up of random electrons would cause anything in the area that receives them, to take on a negative charge, like the infected skin in our experimental ozone bag. For some reason, this negative charge causes germs, etc. to vanish, and rapid healing to take place. WHY? Is it as the hydrogen peroxide proponents say, that free radical oxygen steals electrons away from germs and pathogens, while leaving the normal cells alone?

Interestingly enough, these findings parallel the conclusions of research scientists around the world. Many scientists have proven that men (and animals) function with greater positive vitality in a negatively charged electrical environment.

"Ozone selectively inhibited the growth of human cancer cells."
-Sweet, Kao, et. al. "Science" 1980.

Note: Although I have been unable to find the researcher who did this work, I want to thank "Merlin" for his dedication, and for bringing this information into our awareness.

DOCTOR GERARD SUNNEN

Dr. Gerard Sunnen is Associate Clinical Professor of Psychiatry, New York University, Bellevue Medical Center, New York, NY, 10016. This is a condensation of a discussion I had with Dr. Sunnen on 4/4/88.

Dr. Sunnen is a medical doctor who, after an internship in medicine and surgery, did a mixed residency in psychiatry and neurology. He specializes in biological psychiatry and psychopharmacology. His work, "Ozone in Medicine" is in the section following this one, and his complete references are listed after the article. You may wish to use them for further study. He chose these works after "weeding out" anything he thought might be considered significantly questionable.

STUDIED OZONE IN EUROPE

Dr. Sunnen's interest in ozone dates back to a time when a friend of his had been treated for cancer for five years. The friend decided, because of exasperation with side effects, to stop any further treatments, including surgery, radiation and chemotherapy. This friend of his found out about ozone treatments given in Germany, and asked Dr. Sunnen to investigate their merits. He did this. During his following European trip, Dr. Sunnen visited Dr. R. Viebahn of the Hansler Institute in Illezheim, West Germany, and visited several clinics where he witnessed ozone being applied in the treatment of various clinical conditions, often in an adjunctive capacity.

"WINDOW"

He found a main point, stressed by the Germans, is, that ozone seems to have a "therapeutic window". Patients receive ozone blood treatments in a range from a few micrograms to 100 per milliliter. Any less is ineffective, any more is possibly damaging to the normal cells, (due to their being injured by lipid peroxidation). Also, at the suggested dosages, they don't always "cure" the diseases, but do find that they are halting any further progression or deterioration.

EUROPEANS FAVOR GRADUAL INCREASE

Dr. Sunnen states that Europeans prefer to give the treatments by starting slowly with low dosages, and increasing the concentrations gradually over the long term. They believe low dosages stimulate the immune system best, and that too much actually inhibits it. Americans tend toward advocating higher dosages, and giving them more often, with the intent of directly killing viruses. An analogy to this might be: the use of antibiotics to kill bacteria, where too many antibiotics will also kill off the friendly acidophilus bacteria that our intestines need for digestion. I think that by keeping the "therapeutic window" idea in mind, we should all call for more testing and documentation.

We need to develop a method of determining, on an individual basis, what the level is that would produce maximum viral kill without any damage to healthy tissues.

WHY NO NEWS MENTION

Why don't we hear about this on the news? First, it's not known exactly under what conditions it works best. We don't know if ozone would be outrightly curative in some viral illnesses, but it might be a "softer" therapeutic agent, especially in AIDS and other diseases that lie dormant and then come out. In these cases, known as viremic episodes, viruses exist in the body quietly, and suddenly explode into the system. We don't know why this is, but it is at this point (in the life cycle of the virus) where ozone and other oxygenation therapies may cut down on the population of circulating viruses drastically, purifying the blood.

Ozone therapy can be especially useful in relapses, or exacerbations of viral illnesses like; Herpes, AIDS, even the flu. They all have viremic episodes.

AMOUNT OF INFORMATION OVERWHELMS REPORTERS AND DOCTORS

Why haven't we heard more about oxygenation therapies like ozone? There have been so many documented instances where ozone therapy can be used, that an overwhelming amount of information has been created, and therefore not pursued systematically. We need further research on a few of the more important uses to start with. An American doctor looking at the whole spectrum, the "rainbow", of conditions that the Europeans say ozone offers therapeutic possibilities to, may say this is the pattern of a panacea, and may unjustly respond negatively. It also encompasses a "whole systems viewpoint", rather than the viewpoint of symptom relief, a viewpoint which might be unfamiliar to some. We also might be facing the over-zealousness of some proponents making it easy for detractors to impugn the whole subject.

PUBLIC MISINFORMED

Another recognition problem is within the public mass consciousness. Ozone has been likened to some foreign element floating around covering the globe, or as a poison in smog. The only association people have with it is that it is toxic, or an irritant.

Actually, ozone is a natural product, which, by surrounding the planet, makes our lives possible, by filtering out burning rays; and smog is created by chemical pollutants reacting to it trying to oxidize them. The problem is the pollutants, not the ozone. Ozone, like any drug, can reach a level where you get too much, and it becomes toxic. The dosage is harmful, not the chemical. Too much of anything isn't good for you; and ozone, like any other therapeutic agent, has it's own window of biologically healing properties.

DR. SUNNEN'S PAPER ON HISTORICAL AND CURRENT OZONE USAGE

What follows is a summary of Dr. Sunnen's study "Ozone in Medicine: Overview And Future Directions", which was published in The Journal of Advancement In Medicine, Human Science Press, NY, Fall 88. I have paraphrased it using more common language, and left out some of the involved technical aspects for easier reading. In this form, it is not meant as a medical text, and anyone wishing such a version should contact Dr. Sunnen. The numbers in parentheses (X) refer to the references found at the end of the paper.

INTRODUCTION

We know ozone best from it's role in filtering out the sun's harmful rays. Before 1900, ozone was known to kill bacteria. By WW1, it was used to treat wounds and infections, but without modern generators and plastics technology, the application was difficult. These application problems have been solved by modern technology.

HISTORY OF OZONE

In 1785 Martinus Van Marum noted it's odor and oxidating properties. In 1840 Schonbein named it ozone, from the Greek "ozein", meaning odorant (46). Many have worked on it since, describing and classifying it (42).

In the latter part of the nineteenth century, ozone was found to oxidize certain organic compounds, and interact with double bonds. Using these properties, Harries discovered the structure of natural rubber (42).

Because ozone can destroy toxic or foul smelling pollution, as well as bacteria in sewage, Wiesbaden (W. Germany) began purifying drinking water with it in 1901. Now, Zurich (Switzerland), Florence (Italy), Brussels (Belgium), Marseille (France), Singapore, Moscow, and other major cities do the same.

Kleinman used it to study bacteria. Payr (41), Fisch and Wolff (65) pioneered its use in their clinics, and J. Hansler developed one of the first reliable ozone generators (42,50).

Oxygen atoms exist in several forms:

O, A free atom that's unstable and will react readily.

O_2, Oxygen - colorless as a gas, and pale blue as a liquid.

O_3, Ozone - blue as a gas, and dark blue as a solid, is a powerful oxidant.

O_4, A very unstable, pale blue gas which readily turns into two molecules of oxygen (O_2). There are even higher forms.

98

It is important to note that ozone interacts with tissue and blood. This is the method generally used in ozone therapy. Remove the patient's blood, mix it with ozone, and return it to him. This mixture reacts with the fatty (lipid) structures, and forms lipid peroxides.

There are a number of lipid (fat based) components in whole blood. Among these are: cholesterol, phospholipids, triglycerides, and freefatty acids. Ozone can react with all of these, creating many different end products (16,50). Our bodies buffer this lipid peroxidation with vitamin E, uric acid (33), and enzymes such as S.O.D. (superoxide dismutase), catalase, and the glutathione peroxidase system (36).

The main compounds derived from the lipid peroxidtion are, free radicals, singlet oxygen, hydrogen peroxide, hydroperoxides, hydroperoxide ozonides, carbonyls, alkanes, and alkenes. The hydroperoxides attack viruses, and then in turn are broken down into alcohols by the enzyme glutathione peroxidase.

OZONE APPLICATION

In 1915, A. Wolff (64) is credited with using ozone as a local treatment for wounds. The cups and bags used to apply it were made from natural rubber. They broke down too quickly, causing ozone to fall into disuse. Our modern Teflon and other plastics last much longer, and deliver more precise dosages. For example, a burn area can now be treated without touching the site through use of an ozone inflated bag.

Ozone is used on wounds, burns, staph infections, fungul and radiation injuries, herpes, and gangrene. The dosage is tailored for each condition. A treatment lasts from 3 to 20 minutes, and the concentrations vary from 10 to 80 ug per milliliter. The maximum is 5 parts ozone to 95 parts oxygen. High concentrations are used for disinfection and cleaning, and low concentrations promote skin growth and healing.

In 1935, Payr (41), and Aubourg in 1936 (2) introduced ozone into the rectum, and by this method treated colitis and fistulae. This method is now used in hemorrhoids and anal infections. It promotes healing, and the balance of friendly bacterial cultures.

As an example; for colitis, it is applied daily in increasingly higher concentrations until equilibrium is reached. Then the dosages are lowered in subsequent treatments to promote healing. This method may be found to be optimum in AIDS related bowel infections.

MAJOR BLOOD TREATMENTS

Major Blood treatments are also known as autohemotherapy (AHT). 50 to 100 milliliters of blood are drawn out of the patient, mixed with the ozone/ oxygen mixture, and reintroduced into the body. This produces oxygenation, kills viruses, and enhances circulation. We do not know exactly how it affects all

99

the body systems, or how long it remains. Some people have reported being able to faintly taste ozone after it's reintroduction. Blood ozone treatments have been used to treat virus infections, including: AIDS, hepatitis, flu, some cancers, diabetes, and arteriosclerosis (20,46,44,66). More exacting studies need to be done. Some patients report feelings of well being after ozone treatments, lasting from a few minutes to a few hours.

MINOR BLOOD TREATMENTS

This method involves drawing 10 milliliters of venous blood, mixing it with ozone/oxygen and injecting it into the muscles. This method has treated asthma, acne, and some allergies.

INTRAVENOUS TREATMENT

Now rarely used, this method of direct injection (without first mixing the blood with ozone outside the body), was used by Lacoste in 1951 (27) on gangrene. It is rarely used because of the potential of accidents due to too rapid an injection. He found that up to 10ml of pure ozone/oxygen could be directly injected into the leg artery, or a vein, without getting dangerous bubbles in the blood, since both gases are readily soluble in blood (46).

MUSCULAR INJECTION

Used with blood treatment, this is an added cancer therapy. Up to 10 ml of the pure mixture is injected into the muscles.

OZONATED WATER

Ozone is about 10 times more soluble in water than oxygen. Used mostly in dental surgery, it improves the local oxygen supply, and inhibits bacteria. Ozone water has also been used on peridontal disease, swallowed for treatment of gastric cancer, and applied as a wash in intestinal or bladder inflammation.

OZONE OINTMENTS

Mixed with olive oil, this mixture gives a low strength, long term dose of ozone and lipid peroxidases to the tissues. Used on fungal growths and skin ulcers.

OZONE BATHS

Ozone bubbled through warm water irrigates the skin, to disinfect and treat eczema and skin ulcers.

BLOOD PURIFICATION

An exciting possibility (65,62), all the world's blood supplies may possibly be made viral free! Treating 500 ml of whole blood with 100ml of ozone/oxygen mixture (40-50 ug/ml) is reported to render it virus free without injuring any healthy cells. One particular study (62) tested ten thousand treated samples and found no hepatitis. In the future, this technique may also be used in removing the AIDS virus. One preliminary unpublished study indicates this to be so.

EFFECTS OF OZONE

Most studies, up to this point, have only focused on proving how breathing ozone was toxic, or name it as air pollution. Pure ozone, applied in the proper way, is quite a different story. The studies where animals have inhaled it do not equal the response of the human lungs, because there are so many differences in anatomy and physiology. Mice have the most trouble with it (37), and birds the least (8). Inhaling very low dosages (3) increases enzyme activity, while overdosage can result in bleeding in the lungs. We see again the window concept, and refer you to what "Merlin" found out.

Due to the danger of breathing in too much ozone, modern treatment machines are designed to prevent any leakage into the treatment room, as well as catalytically converting excess ozone to oxygen during administration. Some studies, however, point to a beneficial effect of low dosage ambient ozone (12,63).

BACTERICIDAL, VIRUCIDAL, and FUNGICIDAL ACTION

We have known ozone kills and inhibits pathogens since the nineteenth century. What we haven't done is the tests proving exactly why it has these effects. Only a few micrograms per liter provide germ killing action. It works even faster on viruses than bacteria, at lower dosages, and is influenced by pH, temperature, and other nearby organic compounds.

Different viruses have different susceptibility to destruction by ozone (47,48). for example, the polio virus is forty times more resistant than other viruses.

Ozone's popular reputation as a bactericide centers on it's ability to destroy the pathogen's outer fatty/protein shell (39). In one study (23) it actually penetrated the cell's membrane and changed the DNA. Higher organisms have enzymes that can restabilize disrupted DNA & RNA, where lower forms do not. This could be why ozone, at proper levels, will kill a virus (a lower lifeform), and leave a person's (higher lifeform) cells unharmed.

One study showed the ability to destroy candida fungi to be dependent on their stage of growth (30). Budding cells were the most sensitive. Another study showed a low dose increasing the growth of two other fungi (31).

Viruses are genetic parasites, and can be separated into families, based on structure. Those containing lipids are the most sensitive: herpes, mumps, measles, flu, rabies, HIV/AIDS. In some, the shell is damaged, in others they remain whole, but unable to reproduce. Often the ozone is used up in a blood reaction, and the products of that reaction cause the destruction or inactivation of the pathogens. Although unlikely to be an outright curative by itself, when combined with other therapies, ozone may lessen clinical severity or duration (66,62,29).

101

OZONE AND CANCER

Cancer cells have disturbed metabolisms. Nobel Prize winner Dr. Otto Warburg, in 1925, found cancer cells to function best in the absence of oxygen, in effect, living on fermentation rather than respiration (59). Some authors (56,45) report that tumor cells don't have enough of the proper enzymes (catalase and peroxidase) to resist ozone's actions. One study (51), exposed lung, breast, and uterine cancer cells, alongside normal cells, to ozone over an 8 day period. At .3ppm the cancer growth was inhibited by 40%. .5ppm yielded a 60% inhibition. .8ppm increased it to 90%, and at this level the normal cells showed the first signs of change, slowing activity by 50%. These researchers postulate that cancer cells can't resist the oxidation effects of ozone due to a less functional glutathione system.

Many people have reported ozone's beneficial effects on cancers (45,56,61,66,67), but there is too little controlled data at this time. Several researchers used ozone along with radiation or chemotherapy (53).

MANUFACTURING OZONE

Most medical ozone is produced by passing clinical oxygen through high voltage tubes of 4,000 to 14,000 volts. Since a useful amount only lasts 45 minutes, it must be used immediately. Agricultural concerns produce it by passing air over a special ultraviolet light (185 nanometer wavelength). Never let ether mix with ozone. It is said ozone should not be used (45) when intoxicated, following a recent heart attack, after recent bleeding, during pregnancy, hyperthyroidism, or thrombosis and if the patient shows ozone allergy.

SUMMARY

The use of ozone as a healing agent is being explored, and used in clinical practice, because it manifests bactericidal, virucidal and fungicidal actions. These properties make this high energy molecule very attractive in modern usage. It has only been recently that we have had the technology to properly use it. A lot of experience has been gathered on it's use and proper dosage, mostly in Europe. It has been used externally as a gas, in a solution, and mixed into blood.

A large body of literature exists describing ozone's use on diseases, infections, burns, dental, intestinal, and possibly circulatory conditions. More studies will have to be made concerning:
1. The by-products formed from ozone's use.
2. The purification of stored blood.
3. The inhibition of cancers.
4. The inactivation or repression of viral diseases, especially Herpes and HIV /AIDS.

Remember, *ozone stimulates the immune system in low concentrations, and inhibits it at higher concentrations.*

REFERENCES

SUPPLIED BY DR. SUNNEN TO DOCUMENT HIS OZONE PAPER

1. Akey D, Walton T: Liquid-phase study of ozone inactivation of Venezuelan Equine encephalomyelitis virus. Appl and Environ Microbiol 1985; 50(4):882
2. Aubourg P: L'Ozone medical: Production, Posologie, Modes d'applications cliniques. Bull Med Soc Med Paris 1938; 52:745-749
3. Basset D, Bowen-Kelly E: Rat lung metabolism after 3 days of continuous exposure to 0.6 parts-per-million ozone. Am J Physiol 1986; 250 (2 Part 1):E131-E136
4. Bolton DC, Zee YC, Osebold JW: The biological effects of ozone on representative members of five groups of animal viruses. Environmental Research 1982; 27:476-482
5. Bretscher M: The molecules of the cell membrane. Scientific American 1985 Oct; 253(4):100-110
6. Buckley RD, Hackney JD, Clark K, Posin C: Ozone and human blood. Arch Environ Health 1975; 30:40-43
7. Cech T: RNA as an enzyme. Scientific American 1986 Nov; 255(5):64-76
8. Clamann H: Physical and medical aspects of ozone. In: Physics and Medicine of the Atmosphere and Space. John Wiley and Sons 1960; p.151
9. Clemons GK, Wei D: Effect of short-term ozone exposure on endogenous thyroxine levels in thyroidetomized and hypophysectomized rats. Toxicol Appl Pharmacol 1984; 74(1):86-90
10. Coffin D, Gardner D, Holzman R, Wolock F: Influence of ozone on pulmonary cells. Arch Environ Health 1968; 16:633-636
11. De Vita V, Hellman S, Rosenberg S: Cancer principles and Practice of Oncology. Lippincot. 1985
12. Dyas A, Boughton B, Das B: Ozone killing action against bacterial and fungal species: Microbiological testing of a domestic ozone generator. J Clin Pathol (Lond) 1983; 36(10):1102-1104
13. Folinsbee LJ: Effects of ozone exposure on lung function in man: a review. Rev Environ Health 1981; 3:211-240
14. Folinsbee LJ, Bedi JF, Horvath SM: Pulmonary function after 1 hour continuous heavy exercise in 0.21 parts-per-million ozone. J Appl Physiol Respir Environ Exercise Physiol 1984; 57(4):984-988
15. Gallo R: The AIDS virus. Scientific American 1987 Jan; 256(1):46-74
16. Gumulka J, Smith L: Ozonation of cholesterol. J Am Chem Soc 1983; 105(7):1972-1979
17. Hackney J, Linn W, Mohler J, Collier C: Adaptation to short term respiratory effects of ozone in men exposed repeatedly. J Appl Physiol Respirat Environ Exercise Physiol 1977; 43:82-85

18. Hakomori S: Glycosphingolipids. Scientific American 1986 May; 254(5):44-54
19. Hamelin C: Production of single-strand and double-strand breaks in plasmid DNA by ozone. Int J Radiat Oncol Biol Phys 1985; 11(2):253-258 20. Hansler J, Weiss H: Beitrag zum Unterschied swischen HOT und Ozontherapie mit dem Ozonosan. Erfaahr hk 1976; 25:185-188
21. Held P: Verbrennungen. OzoNachrichten 1983; 2:84
22. Howell N, Sager R: Differential effects of mitochondrial inhibitors on normal and tumorigenic mouse cells. Fed Proc 1977; 36:356-360
23. Ihde AJ: The development of modern chemistry. Harper and Row. 1964
24. Ishizaki K, Sawadaishi D, Miura K, Shinriki N: Effect of ozone on plasmid DNA of Escheria coli in situ. Water Res 1987; 21(7):823-828
25. Ivanova O, Bogdanov M, Kazantseva V, Gabrilevskaya L, Kodkind G, Akulov K, Drozdov S: Ozone inactivation of enteroviruses in sewage. Vopr Virusol 1983; 0(6):693-698
26. Katzenelson E, Kletter B, Shuval H: Inactivation kinetics of viruses and bacteria by use of ozone. J Am Water Works Assoc 1974; 66:725-729
27. Kulle TJ, Sauder LR, Hebel JR, Chatham MD: Ozone response relationships in healthy nonsmokers. Am Rev Respir Dis 1985; 132(1):36-41
28. Lacoste. Gaz med de France 1951;315 (Ref. Petersen, Med Kl 53;1958) 2078 29. Lohr A, Gratzek J: Bactericidal and paraciticidal effects of an activated air oxidant in a closed aquatic system. J Aquaric Aquat Sci 1984; 4(4 1/2):1-8
30. Mattassi R, Franchina A, D'Angelo F: Die Ozontherapie als Adjuvans in der Gefaspathologie. OzoNachrichten 1982; 1:2
31. Matus V, Nikava A, Prakopava Z, Konyew S: Effect of ozone on the survivability of Candida utilis cells. Vyestsi AkadNavuk Bssr Syer Biyal Navuk 1981; 0(3):49-52
32. Matus V, Lyskova T, Sergienko I, Kustova A, Grigortsevich T, Konev V: Fungi growth and sporulation after a single treatment of spores with ozone. Mikol Fitopatol 1982; 16(5):420-423
33. Mc Donell W, Horstman D, Abdul-Salaam S, House D: Reproducibility of individual responses to ozone exposure. Am Rev Respir Dis 1985; 131(1):36-40
34. Meadows J, Smith R: Uric acid protection of nucleobases from ozone induced degradation. Arch Biochem Biophys 1986; 246(2):838-845
35. Medical World News. Nov 9 1987
36. Melton CE: Effects of long term exposure to low levels of ozone : A review. Aviation, Space, and Environmental
37. Menzel D: Ozone: an overview of its toxicity in man and animals. Toxicol and Environ Health 1984; 13:183-204
38. Mittler S, King M, Burkhardt B: Toxicity of ozone. AMA Arch Ind Health 1957; 15:191-197
39. Miura K, Veda T, Shinriki N, Ishizaki K, Harada F: Degradation of nucleic acids with ozone. Specific internucleotidic bond cleavage of ozone treated transfer RNA with aniline acetate. Chem Pharm Bull 1984; 32(2):651-657
40. Mudd JB, Leavitt R, Ongun A, McManus T: Reaction of ozone with amino acids and proteins. Atmos Environ 1969; 3:669-682

41. Mustafa M, Lee S: Pulmonary biochemical alterations resulting from ozone exposure. Ann Occup Hyg 1976; 19:17-26
42. Partington JR: A History of Chemistry. Macmillan and Co. 1962
43. Payr E: Uber ozonbehandlung in der chirurgie. Munch med Wschr 1935; 82:220-291
44. Razumovskii SD, Zaikov GE: Ozone and its reactions with organic compounds. Elsevier. 1984
45. Riesser V, Perrich J, Silver B, McCammon J: Possible mechanism of poliovirus inactivation by ozone. In: Forum on Ozone Disinfection. Proceedings of the International Ozone Institute, Syracuse, N.Y. 1977:186-192
46. Rilling S: The basic clinical applications of ozone therapy. Ozonachrichten 1985; 4:7-17
47. Rilling S, Viebahn R: The use of ozone in medicine. 1987. Haug
48. Riva-Sanseverino E: The influence of ozone therapy on the remineralization of the bone tissue in osteoporosis. OzoNachrichten 1987; 6:75-79
49. Rokitansky O: Klinik und biochemie der ozon-therapy. Hospitalis 1982; 52:643 and 711
50. Roy, D, Wong PK, Engelbrecht RS, Chian ES: Mechanism of enteroviral inactivation by ozone. Appl Envir Microbiol 1981; 41:718-723
51. Roy D, Englebrecht R, Chian E: Comparative inactivation of 6 enteroviruses by ozone. Am Water Works Assoc J 1982; 74(12):660-664
52. Schonbein C: Notice of CF Sch., the discoverer of ozone. Annual report of the Board of Regents of the Smithsonian Inst 1868 (Wash.D.C., U.S. Government Printing Office 1869) 185-192
53. Schulz S: Ozonisiertes olivenol-experimentelle ergebnisse der wundheilung am tiermodell. OzoNachrichen 1982; 1:29
54. Smith LL: Cholesterol autoxidation of lipids. Chemistry and Physics of Lipids 1987; 44:87-125
55. Sweet J, Kao MS, Lee D, Hagar W: Ozone selectively inhibits growth of human cancer cells. Science 1980; 209:931-933
56. Takahashi Y, Miura Y: A selective enhancement of xenobiotic metabolizing systems of rat lungs by prolonged exposure to ozone. Environ Res 1987; 42(2):425-434
57. Tietz C: Ozontherapie als adjuvans in der onkologie. OzoNachrichten 1983; 2:4
58. Turk R: Ozone in dental medicine. Ozonachrichten 1985; 4:61-65
59. Van Der Zee J, Tijssen-Christianse K, Dubbelman T, Van Steveninck J: The influence of ozone on human red blood cells: Comparison with other mechanisms of oxidative stress. Biochim Biophys Acta 1987; 924(1):111-118
60. Varro J: Die krebsbehandlung mit ozon. Erfahr hk 1974; 3:178-181
61. Verweij H, Christianse K, Van Stevenick J: Ozone induced formation of O-O-dityrosine cross-links in proteins. Biochim Biophys Acta 1982; 701(2):180-184
62. Viebahn R: The biochemical process underlying ozone therapy. OzoNachrichten 1985; 4:18-30
63. Vogelsberger W, Herget H: Klinische ozonanwendung. OzoNachrichten 1983; 2:1

64. Warburg O: On the origin of cancer cells. Science 1956; 123:309-315
65. Washuttl J, Steiner I, Szalay S: Untersuchungen uber die auswirkungen von ozon auf verschiedene biochemische parameter bei blutproben in vitro. Erfahr hk 1979; 28:766
66. Washuttl J, Viebahn R: Ozonisiertes olivenol-zusammensetzung and desinfizierence wirksamkeit. OzoNachrichten 1982; 1:25
67. Wenzel D, Morgan D: Interactions of ozone and antineoplastic drugs on rat fibroblasts and Walker rat carcinoma cells. Res Commun Chem Pathol Pharmacol 1983; 40(2):279-288
68. Werkmeister H: Subatmospheric O2/O3 treatment of therapy-resistant wounds and ulcerations. OzoNachrichten 1985; 4:53-59
69. Wehrli F: Transact 6 Ham 1957;318
70. Wolcott J, Zee YC, Osebold J: Exposure to ozone reduces influenza disease severity and alters distribution of influenza viral antigens in murine lungs. Appl Environ Microbiol 1982; 443:723-731
71. Wolff A: Eine medizinische verwendbarkeit des ozons. Dtsch Med Wschr 1915;311
72. Wolff H: Das medizinische ozon. VFM Publications. Heidelberg. 1979. 73. Wolff H: Aktuelles in der ozontherapy. Erfarhr hk 1977; 26:193-196
74. Zabel W: Gansheitsbehandlung der geschwulsterkrankungen. Hippokrates 1960; 31:751-760

OZONE VIDEO REVIEW

"What oxygen can't do for you, ozone will."

Here are some introductory remarks from the Hansler ozone generator company's video on ozone. It was supplied to me by Medizone Co. of NY.

Ozone was discovered in 1840, and called "strange stuff".

Used in surgery in the U.S. in 1930's.

Dentist E.A Fish started ozone therapy proper and wrote a lengthy thesis on it.

In the 1950's the problem of precise and reliable ozone application was solved by the pioneering work of chemist and physicist J. Hansler (Hansler corporation, W. Germany), allowing ozone therapy to be widely used in medicine. His multi-patented invention is the very basis of all ozone equipment.

In the Hansler process, medical oxygen flows through two consecutive high tension (4,000 to 14,000 volt) electrical tubes, producing ozone.

Hans Wolfe, in 1979, published the book "Medical Ozone."

TWO GOOD MEDICAL OZONE BOOKS

OZONE IN MEDICAL THERAPY

THE RESULT OF 50 YEARS OF DEVELOPMENT OF OZONE/OXYGEN APPLICATION IN MEDICAL THERAPY

Edited by Julius LaRaus, Chairman - Ozone Medical Technology Committee, International Ozone Association

This valuable new book includes ozone medical papers delivered at the Sixth International Ozone Meeting held in Washington, D.C. in May of 1983, plus a compilation from existing literature of ozone application, showing diseases, and other medical uses, method of application, concentration, and reference literature.

It includes the treatment of viral diseases such as herpes zoster, herpes simplex, hepatitis, circulation problems, cancer research, etc. The book is organized into 14 Main Sections.
The price is $75.00, for IOA members, $80.00 for non members.
Order from International Ozone Association, 83-OT Oakwood Ave., Norwalk, CT 06850.

CONTENTS

THE USE OF OZONE IN MEDICINE
A PRACTICAL HANDBOOK AND REFERENCE GUIDE

Professor Siegfried Rilling, MD, and Renate Viebahn, Ph.D., are two of the foremost ozone therapy practitioners, researchers, and proponents of our time. Based in Germany, their book "The Use of Ozone in Medicine, a Practical Handbook and Reference Guide" is the definitive work on medical ozonation.

"Primarily intended for practical use... the book doesn't focus on history, but provides information on how much of an ozone/oxygen mixture is to be applied in what dosage and using what methods for what indication(s)" "This streamlines the book into a compressed, informative and clear guideline, equipped with indices, lists, tables, and alphabetical reference sections."

It contains references, credits and current work in the field. It is the first English translation referring to: the large body of European ozone knowledge, professionals, seminars, training facilities, organizations and journals. Problems are discussed openly, and physicians, surgeons, dentists, and veterinary specialists are focusing on the new aspects opened up by this publication.

AIDS
AIDS
AIDS

AIDS FACTS

41 million Americans have serious arthritis, 20 million have herpes, 13 million have serious diabetes. Comprehend these numbers. This is 74 million, or <u>over one third of our population</u>, <u>EVERY THIRD PERSON</u> and we've counted only three diseases. We don't think much about negative things, we try to ignore them so we can enjoy life. Really thinking about just one disease is scary enough, but, since ignoring it won't help you and your family, let's look at the scariest one. We'll look at AIDS.

In June of 88, the Stockholm Worldwide Aids Conference announced that:

WORLD
200,000 now have full-blown AIDS
150,000 new cases are expected in 1988
5 -10 million people are carrying the virus
138 countries have reported it

U.S.
64,000 active cases
New case every 14 minutes
1,500,000 people infected
38% of those infected will develop AIDS in 5 - 6 years
The virus can remain undetected in the blood supply
They know of no vaccine within 5 years (?)

U.S. Surgeon General KOOP:

"By 1992, 365,000 will be <u>actively</u> infected."

Two congressmen, who have studied the AIDS problem for years, questioned the statement in the Surgeon General's "Understanding AIDS" pamphlet (mailed to every house in the U.S.) that "You won't get AIDS from a mosquito bite." They were told by his staff that "The surgeon General assumes that you won't hit the mosquito as it bites you." They read this fact into the Congressional Record. Note: Dengue Fever and Malaria are transmitted by mosquitoes.

Doctors in a southern state, a tourist haven, are required by law to report all AIDS cases. A doctor recently stated that he reported 2 cases, then heard, two months later on the news, that there were, "no cases reported in this county...."

A California physician, Dr. Robert Strecker MD, Ph.D., has produced a video showing how the AIDS virus was created/mutated in a lab. He proves that the AIDS virus got 50% of it's genes from bovine lukemia virus, and 50% from sheep visna virus. Dr. Robert B. Strecker, M.D. 1501-OT Colorado Blvd., Los Angeles, CA 90041.

The point I'm making here is that we really don't know just how bad things are, or how fast the disease will spread. You don't know how soon you'll be at risk, no matter what your race, age, or lifestyle. AMA president Dr. John J Courey: "There is no cure (for AIDS)... and no immunization." He also said that each case brings the medical industry another 40 to 150 million dollars per thousand victims. AIDS testing alone is worth billions.

WHAT WE KNOW ABOUT AIDS

AIDS is a virus. A virus works by burrowing in, and attaching itself, to a cell's genetic material. Tough to eradicate inside the cell - without killing everything else along the way.

Hope is coming steadily from the oxygenation proponents. The Medizone Company of NY, states they have: "inactivated the virus" in human blood, stored and living, using ozone autohemotherapy. Compare this fact with this historical statement of Dr. Koch in 1967. Here he is speaking about his oxygenation catalyst therapy (I will tell you more about Dr. William F. Koch, MD, Ph.D., later):

"We can show the profession that never was there a treatment that removed the virus from the host cell once it entered, that is, one and a half minutes after the virus has penetrated, the virus is so tightly bound that no amount of vaccine, immune serum, antitoxin or anything else can accomplish the separation. BUT OUR CHEMISTRY DOES MAKE THE SEPARATION, leaving the host cell in full functional ability while the virus is no longer to be found. And it does not make any difference what the virus is; measles, or rabies, or anything else." (There was no AIDS in 1967)

Later on in this book, we'll see how Dr. Koch's above statement will sound similar to the Medizone ozone research, which shows that the hydroxyperoxide radical, created by ozone infusion, identifies and destroys the virus within infected cells.

WEST GERMAN DOCTOR REMOVES AIDS!

USES COMBINATION OZONE THERAPY!

Address delivered by:
Alexander Preuss
D-700 Stuttgart 1 (West) Physician Bebel Strasse 29
- Private Practice
Federal Republic of Germany
Tel. (0711) 63 49 63

POSITIVE TREATMENT RESULTS IN AIDS THERAPY

In 1982, I faced my first AIDS patient. The patients concerned were always noticeable due to anergy (lack of immune response) of the skin (they looked bad), and, facultatively, due to loss of weight as well as other nonspecific symptoms. In the intensive wards, death generally occurred within (a minimum of) 2 days and a maximum of 3 months. The causes for death were generally sepsis or Pneumocystitis carinii (highly contagious, epidemic, interstitial plasma cell pneumonia), or cytomegalovirus. This course of events I was able to observe up to the end of 1984. AIDS did not become a special challenge to me, however, until a former student friend with a positive HTLV III test came to me for consultation.

As it is known that the actual disease(s) occurring through AIDS consists of a combination of viral, fungal and bacterial infections, I searched for a substance which is virucidal, fungicidal and bactericidal at the same time. Ozone was here the obvious solution, as this was a substance which has been in use for many decades for the elimination of microorganisms.

On account of the origins of retrovirus and the immune defect resulting from it, I applied the following combination therapy:

1) Suramin (transcriptase inhibitor)
2) **Ozone**
3) Immunomodulation
4) Substitution of basic systems (minerals, vitamins)
5) Hygienization of the intestinal flora.

Under this therapy, ***immediate improvement of conditions occurred in the AIDS patients***. Other infection conditions present at the same time, such as e.g. hepatitis B or gastrointestinal candidiasis disappeared automatically within 5-10 days.

As based on my experience, the following tests are necessary where the presence of AIDS is suspected:

1) HTLV III antibody test through ELISA,
   and, when this is positive, followed by:
2) Immunoblot and HTLV III antibody test via IFT, then:
3) Stamp test for skin anergy, and:
4) Screening of essential minerals,
5) Vitamin screening, and
6) Examination of feces for dysbacteria.

In my opinion, skin anergy forms the boundary symptom between the initial and the advanced stages of AIDS, it being the first symptom of AIDS as a manifest disease. If skin anergy is present, the intestinal flora is then generally coated with funguses in most cases, so that dysbacteria are present.

Up to now, skin anergy has always been accompanied by a deficiency of vitamins and minerals.

The skin anergy is followed by oropharyngeal candidiasis, fungus-infected seborrheal eczema and brown-reddish efflorescences on the bending side of the arms and trunk.

According to experience up till now, the onset of skin anergy can be followed any time by fatal sepsis.

CASE HISTORIES

CASE 1: Early symptoms:
   1) Chronic sinusitis
   2) Fungus-infected seborrheal eczema
   3) Dysbacteria (disturbance of intestinal flora)
   4) Vitamin deficiency
   5) Mineral deficiency
   6) Dermic anergy.

The patient refused the AIDS test based on the reasoning as to "how could he ever catch such a disease?". Five months later, acute concomitant dermatomyositis under the aspect of two viral infections, the one being hepatitis B and the other a subsequently detected HTLV III infection, were evidenced. Candida Ag was found in the patient's serum. Five days after starting the above combination therapy, laboratory chemical tests showed that the initial hepatitis B had completely disappeared, and serum Candida Ag was negative after 10 days. *Subsequent history: the patient has been fully capable of work and clinically healthy since treatment. HTLV III antibodies have further increased, thus indicating a good immune status. No further therapy is being applied at present.*

CASE 2: Early Symptoms:
   1) Rapid growth of multiple warts on the back of both hands
   2) Mineral deficiency
   3) Vitamin deficiency
   4) Chronic pancreatitis
   5) Skin anergy.

HTLV III was positive. After applying combination therapy, the warts disappeared within a few days and have not recurred since. According to his own report, he had never felt so well in years. *Subsequent history: the patient has been fully capable of work and clinically healthy since treatment. HTLV III antibodies have further increased, thus indicating a good immune status. No further therapy is being applied at present.*

CASE 3: Early Symptoms:
1) Apparent Pfeiffer's disease 2 years previously
2) Intermittent occurrence of adynami-crises (tot. exhaustion)
3) Vitamin deficiency
4) Mineral deficiency
5) Lues II
6) Chronic pancreatitis
7) Recurrent oropharyngeal candidiasis
8) Dysbacteria (disturbance of intestinal flora)
9) Dermic anergy.

The patient initially refused the AIDS test as he was afraid of discrimination due to obligatory registration with the Health Administration. Thus three months passed unattended. The patient was then admitted to hospital for a highly feverish infection with profuse attacks of diarrhea, upon which gastrointestinal candidiasis was found. At the same time, a polyneuritis of all extremities occurred. Systematic antimycotic therapy was carried out. Following dismissal from hospital, the patient came to me on account of the polyneuritis. This was caused to disappear within 3 days applying homoeopathics, following which general well-being was reported. Eight days later, there were renewed adynamic crises, oropharyngeal candidiasis and the sudden recurrence of reddish-brown efflorescences on the bending side of the arms and the trunk. A combination therapy was started. Already on the following day, the patient felt well and started work once more. *Subsequent history: since then, the patient has been fully capable of work and clinically healthy since treatment. The skin efflorescences disappeared. No further therapy is being considered at present.*

CASE 4: The patient appeared with AIDS already diagnosed. He had apparently been HTLV positive since 1983, and had been under treatment at a university clinic. A skin anergy was diagnosed in 1984. For one year previously he had been suffering from chronic diarrhea, depressions, thoughts of suicide, disturbed concentration and a pronouncedly deficient short-term memory. As regards his profession, he had not been able to work since this time. The physician in his confidence had occasionally issued statements testifying him incapable of work due to illness: however, he had been totally incapable of working for 4 months at the time he sought consultation. Neither at the university clinic nor with his physician had any form of therapy been initiated. From external evidence, a considerable change in personality had taken place in the course of 1 year. Over the last year, he had also twice been obliged to take systemic antimycotics due to a severe hoarseness.

Whole-body examination was immediately carried out and yielded the following diagnoses:

1) Cortical cerebral atrophy
2) Thrush (candidiasis of the buccal mucous membranes)
3) Vitamin deficiency
4) Mineral deficiency

The combination therapy was carried out. The chronic diarrhea and the thrush instantly disappeared, the general condition clearly improved. As to the development of the cortical cerebral atrophy within the context of AIDS, the outcome cannot yet be determined. *The patient is once more capable of work.*

CASE 5: The patient appeared with the diagnosis of suspected AIDS pronounced by himself. He himself had been witness to four of his former sexual partners dying of the disease since 1983. He had not been able to decide in favor of an AIDS test as, in his opinion, no therapy is conducted in the university hospitals and, instead, the AIDS patients are simply nursed until they die. Previous diseases: gonorrhea, lung tuberculosis, fatty liver due to chronic alcoholism (no longer a problem, since 10 years ago) lues II, herpes genitalis, chronic persistent hepatitis, and recurrent infections of the urinary tract. The AIDS test, which was carried out immediately, was positive in all 3 test results. In addition, skin anergy was found. Further tests produced the following diagnoses:

1) Tinea nasolabialis on both sides
2) Vitamin deficiency
3) Mineral deficiency

Combination therapy was carried out. *The patient now continues to be fully capable of working.*

The AIDS patients I treated were aged between 22 and 48. All are sexually active as before. Up till now, after application of the combination therapy, no communication of the HTLV III infection to sexual partners could be demonstrated.

As a result of these good treatment results, this form of AIDS therapy ought to be carried out as soon as possible after the HTLV III infection. A positive AIDS test in all 3 testing procedures represents the absolute indication for this therapy.

The most attractive aspect of this combination therapy is the fact that *it is completely unimportant as to whether a virus, fungus or bacterium underlies the AIDS infection. Even if AIDS should be an autoimmune disease, this therapy is effective simply because it is non-specific and covers all possible causes.*

As there is a certain similarity between AIDS and cancer, I would also attempt this form of therapy in cancer on account of its being non-specific. Ladies and Gentlemen, as long as medical science is not yet in a position to provide an effective therapy for AIDS, I consider this form of therapy as being a method of choice in combating AIDS. Thank you for your kind attention.

VIRUSES

In each reproducing cell in our bodies are two substances, RNA and DNA, the "helix" form discovered by Crick and Watson. They contain the genetic blueprint for the cell, and the whole body. Viruses aren't cells, they are either DNA or RNA genetic material, but not both, and surrounded by a coat of protein. Since they have only half of the genetic material, they cannot reproduce on their own. They multiply by attaching themselves to the inner DNA or RNA of normal cells, taking it over and forcing the cell to make more of the virus. Picture slave labor. They wait there, and emerge when our defenses are down. Evil sounding, aren't they?

Outside of a host cell, they are pretty inert. So, how can oxygenation stop them if they are hiding in the cells?

To spread, a virus must travel. Every cell is immersed in bodily fluids, mostly the intercellular fluid. If the intercellular fluids have all the oxygen compounds, enzymes, peroxides, minerals, electrolysis processes and compounds, etc. that they need, as in an optimum health situation, then the virus might have a hard time leaving it's host cell and moving out to infect another.

The Medizone people and the 3000 German doctors who have all announced that they have, before, and can continue, to kill AIDS and other viruses with ozone, explain that the diseased cells have lowered titers (concentrations or strengths) of their enzymatic coatings. Because of this, the hydroxyperoxides and other free radical scavengers created by blood ozonation identify and destroy diseased cells only. They state that to get them all, they must give the patient repeated applications of ozone.

Looking at a diseased cell electrochemically, the first thing that differentiates it, from normal cells, is the protein coating that surrounds it. It is different, contoured distinctly. Since the virus is a parasite, it is drawing off the cellular electricity or life force of the host cell. The host cell, having to give up it's life force to the parasite, doesn't have enough of it's own. This is a condition of cell stress, and any protein coat manufactured under these conditions would be substandard. The infected cell protein coating is weak, dilute, not at full strength, or, in other words, evidences a "lowered titer".

Nature's immune system and it's cells, if not blocked, can identify and attack these invaders, even within itself. This is because they've not all "gone bad".

"RESEARCHERS HOPE TO TEST OZONE IN BLOOD AS TREATMENT FOR AIDS"

- Headline - The Washington Times, April 30, 1987.

"OZONE MAY HELP VICTIMS OF AIDS"
"STUDIES FIND OZONE MAY FIGHT AIDS VIRUS"
"OZONE MAY BECOME AIDS TREATMENT"
"TESTS FIND OZONE MAY CURB AIDS SYMPTOMS"
"OZONE MAY AID TREATMENT OF AIDS"

- Headlines announcing New England Journal of Medicine study, by Dr. Kenneth Wagner. Released Oct. 27th, 1988.

MEDIZONE, THE U.S. MEDICAL OZONE CO.

Medizone, 2B-OT, 123 E. 54th St.
New York, NY 10022

Terrence McGrath, CEO & President
William Gregory, Sales Manager

NEWS MEDIA SILENCE

By all rights, the story of Medizone's treatment methods should be announced all over our national news media soon. Major news providers say, they will not report on any new treatments, no matter how good they sound, until human testing is approved by the FDA. Many drugs have, however, been widely announced before such approval. Medizone is diligently supplying all the studies and tests necessary, to get FDA human test approval. Medizone is also human testing in foreign countries, as well as seeking human test approval in other major countries. *I wrote the above paragraph, in the summer of 1988, since then, the announcement has been made, that the Veterans Administration has done their own testing, using rectal insufflation of ozone on AIDS patients. Their success was picked up by the national news media. The VA is not under the FDA jurisdiction, so they didn't need permission to do the studies. Medizone and the Veterans Administration, are said to be looking into working together, in a VA hospital in New York.*

EUROPEAN TREATMENT HISTORY

The same ozone treatment as that used by Medizone, has already proven, within the proper procedures, to be safe, effective, and 100% non-toxic, in over 30 years of human application by thousands of European physicians.

FDA APPROVAL NEEDED

The only snag in using it on more than the veterans, in other words, the general public, is waiting for FDA approval. Medizone's U.S. approval process has taken, so far, over 3 years. During this time, Medizone has submitted to the FDA: 982 slides, the 11 Dr. Preussch ancedotal German case histories of AIDS cures (see previous section), and performed numerous flawless animal, and cell non-toxicity studies in highly accredited labs. The FDA keeps sending them back to do more studies. The VA went ahead and did their own testing. By the way, two of the Medizone board members are former FDA officials: Dr. Garvey, who was in charge of submissions to the FDA, and Dr. Goddard, who was head of the FDA.

TYPE OF OZONE

Medizone's Ozone, produced from pure oxygen, is a combination of polyatomic oxygen - O_3, O_4, O_{5+}, etc., forms. The ozone is produced by treating pure oxygen with ultraviolet light at about 185 nanometer wavelengths.

HOW MEDIZONE OZONE WORKS

In Medizone's proposed blood ozonation process, ozone never enters the body. Blood is withdrawn and exposed to the highly reactive, pure oxygen produced, medical ozone. This interface starts an immediate chemical reaction with the blood. The ozone combines with blood lipids and forms a chain process called "Lipid Peroxidation" which, combining with water, creates hydroxy peroxides. These are free radical scavengers. These free radicals attack weakened cells - cells with a weakened chemistry and/or electrical charge from viral infection.

VIRUSES LOWER ENZYME LEVELS

When an invading virus incorporates itself into a cell, it reduces the cellular enzyme "titer" (strength level). The free radicals, that were formed by the ozone's interface with the blood, react with the long molecular chains, and find the cells with the lowered enzyme levels, the weakened links. Please refer to Dr. Sunnen's article in a previous section for a more complete technical understanding of this process.

AN UNSCIENTIFIC EXPLANATION OF THE MEDIZONE PROCESS

I will digress now and try to explain it in an admittedly unscientific manner: ozone is exposed to the patient's blood outside his body. Usually in a hypodermic syringe, and shaken. This exposure immediately uses up the ozone, and creates a complex set of compounds called the "blood drug product". The whole chemical reaction is called a "lipid peroxide reaction". The created compounds combine with water and form our beneficial free radical agents called "hydroxyperoxides".

These free radical agents and the blood they're in, are put back into the bloodstream, and travel through it to all the body parts. Along the way, it's electrically being ignored by normal cells, or attracted by diseased ones. This is like checking out all the cells of the body, while scavenging for damaged (diseased) cells. The hydroxy peroxide free radicals can do this, due to an interesting ability they possess. Because of their electrical and chemical makeup, they are only attracted to weak cells, and therefore attack only the ones with viruses inside them.

118

HOW OZONE "CHOOSES" THE DISEASED CELLS

Ozone's by-products have this selectivity because they are the attractive opposites of diseased cells. Cells infected with a virus have a weakened vitality, which shows up as lowered levels of enzyme activity. A free radical hydroxyperoxide sees the diseased cell's low enzyme level as an enemy "flag" and attacks it.

On a metaphysical level, we could also speculate that an infected cell is weakened due to the disease drawing off it's "Life Force". If that sounds too cosmic for you, might I again refer you to the work of the biochemist and two time Nobel Prize recipient Dr. Otto Warburg, who stated that cancer resulted from a chronic *lack of energy* in the normal cell.

Because of the "survival instinct" programmed into every living thing, the cells still try to manufacture their enzymes, even under the stress of the parasitic virus invasion. But, since the genetic codes of the viruses have attached themselves to, and altered the cells, the cells can't do a good job of manufacturing their enzymes.

These diseased cells with lowered enzyme levels aren't complete, and therefore are seeking to balance themselves by interacting with the free radical hydroxy peroxides, which by themselves are also unstable. Both seeking balance, they join together in their eventual mutual destruction and elimination, benefiting the patient.

NORMAL CELLS UNTOUCHED

Normal, healthy cells aren't lacking for vitality, and don't react with the free radical agents. They have strong, balanced enzymes that, in a sense, make them "invisible". They are complete, and not receptive to reacting.

The obvious beauty of this, is that the by-products of the ozone process "target" diseased cells. Repeated treatments are necessary because viruses seem to be more susceptible at different stages of their growth, and as an ozone reaction winds down, a new one must be introduced to react with any viruses left over from the previous treatment.

VIRUS DETECTION

Still today, even with our modern technology, you can't easily identify a virus sitting/hiding inside a genetic complex. It's very difficult to do. So, how are you going to prove you're going in and doing anything to it, if you can't even find it? This fact has lead to a lot of confusion, and more research needs to be done on methods of detection. The subjective evidence of ozone treated AIDS patients having "health" returning still piles up, however, so *something* is going on.

HYDROGEN PEROXIDE AND MEDIZONE OZONE TREATMENTS COMPARED

Medizone's president, Mr. McGrath, suspects that Hydrogen Peroxide ingestion is a totally different chemical process than using intravenous ozone. Ozone, unlike hydrogen peroxide, does not raise the PO2 level (a sampled difference in oxygen levels, when comparing the arterial and venous systems), unless administered rectally.

Also, the Medizone company, at first, will not put ozone directly into the body. The Europeans and Mexican clinics occasionally inject it, but problems might arise through too rapid an injection.

Further, the Medizone process is not a direct method of action like hydrogen peroxide. It is *a totally reactive process*. This means that when introduced into the blood, it creates a reaction, it is *the reaction* that does the work of creating beneficial free radicals to inactivate viruses. The ozone disappears almost immediately, at the start of the reaction.

OZONE IS AFFORDABLE

According to the AMA's president; from diagnosis to death, each AIDS patient costs $140,000 in medical care, plus $10,000 to $15,000 is spent per year for AZT. This is a large financial drain on patients and insurance companies. Medizone ozone therapy will cost approximately $3,500 for 21 daily consecutive treatments.

MEDIZONE - THE COMPANY

Medizone's modern offices are situated just off 5th AVE., in New York City. I had a meeting, and a number of conversations, with Terrence McGrath, the President of Medizone. He was kind enough to supply me with a technical description of his Medizone process. These technical details are reproduced for you, in a copy of his letter to me, at the end of this section. Something for everyone.

YOUNG COMPANY

Medizone, formed in March of 1986, is a young company in the midst of delicate negotiations with many financial concerns and governmental agencies in many countries. For this reason, the information I have to give you is only a current "snapshot" of events. Some of this information might be outdated by the time you read this. Future editions of this book will reflect any changes as they occur.

MEDIZONE'S PRESIDENT

Terrence O. McGrath, Medizone's founder and president, brings a wealth of scientific knowledge to his enterprise, having served in the British military as a lecturer on bacteriological warfare. He describes himself in almost humble terms, but has a strong character and sense of what's right. He wouldn't let me photograph him, and states "Ozone is the real story, not me." and, "I'm only bringing to market the work of the brilliant pioneers in this

120

field, who went unnoticed by the medical community and are mostly all deceased.".

He and I share the sentiment that it is best to do something for the benefit of humanity, but we also know that many brilliant ideas have been lost through a lack of correct marketing techniques. Medizone is bringing Ozone Therapy into the mainstream of U.S. medical thinking, through an exhaustive and time consuming process of carefully documented medical laboratory studies.

MEDIZONE'S PATENT AND FINANCES

Medizone has a patent, #4,632,980, and FDA I.N.D. (Investigative New Drug) status, which gives them sole rights to: "The use of ozone in the inactivation of lipid envelope viruses within blood and blood products that may be returned to a mammalian host". The patent has been issued in the U.S., and is being processed in other countries as well. This patent covers ozone's use, both inside and outside of the body. In effect, they have the medical ozone market "sewn up" here.

As far as their financial position is concerned, they are a public corporation. Their stock sells "over the counter" (OTC) and is currently listed on the "Pink Sheets", at about 50 cents. They have about 32 market makers listed in the Pink Sheets, and their stock can be purchased by anyone. One of the market makers is Ross Bottomly, at Alpine Securities, 440 East 400 South, Suite 200-OT, Salt Lake City , Utah 84111, 800/274-5588, or 800/521-5588.

They are planning to market the Hansler (West German) ozone producing machines in the U.S., and they intend to market the ozone drug "Medizone". In this proposed arrangement, medical doctors would be licensed to have the Medizone producing machines in their treatment rooms, and be charged for each dosage generated. Medizone plans to acquire 51% of the stock of the Hansler ozone generator company in West Germany.

MEDIZONE"S WORLD MARKET POTENTIAL

Medizone is opening up operations around the world. The United Kingdom, Australia, Singapore, and Canadian operations are all moving steadily toward government approval and completed business arrangements. For example, Medizone has formed a company in Canada, Medizone (Canada) Ltd. ("MCL"), and elected a board of directors with David Mellnick, Chairman. He's a "Queens Counsellor" an honored lawyer. They are now working on funding, lines of distribution, marketing, etc. The human testing submissions are being made to the HPB (Health Preservation Bureau - Canada's version of the FDA).

Medizone has set a priority on securing rights in these world markets, and plans on entering the European Economic Community as soon as possible. The British operation is a wholly owned subsidiary of Medizone in NY. The U.K. medical people are requiring two animal toxicity studies before granting human testing approval.

In Canada, Medizone set up their Canadian operation, and then sold 20% of it to local interests. Canada has it's own medical approval system through the CHPB, and approval is being vigorously pursued there as well. In Bangkok and Singapore, the parent company, Medizone/NY, will probably own a minority position. They have deduced that with the differences in customs and language, it is best to let them "row their own boat". It is hoped that Medizone will be commercial there by the end of 1988. All protocols done there will be at the standard FDA levels. Hard to ignore.

In Australia, they just met with financiers interested in being the partners in Medizone - Australia.

In a new development, Medizone just trained an American doctor in the Medizone treatment process, and has sent him, with two donated ozone machines, and their sales manager, to Zaire. Zaire has a runaway AIDS epidemic, 40% of the population. They will use ozone immediately on 100 people there, 50 youngsters, and 50 Adults. They are not going to waste time with testing something that's been in use for 30 years in Europe.

PUNDITS EXCITED

"Confidential:Report from Zurich", "Penny Stock Insider", and "Low Priced Stock Edition" (stock market advisory newsletters) are urging their readers to get in on Medizone now, comparing the opportunity to getting in on Xerox, IBM, or Polaroid when they were unknown.

LARGE SCOPE OF FUTURE MEDIZONE APPLICATIONS

While completing the FDA approval process and pursuing the world markets, Medizone is also looking ahead at new applications for ozone. For example, preliminary research has led them to considering skin application of Medizone. At the same time, they have temporarily given up on ozone baths, stating that too much ozone is lost to the atmosphere by the bath method for medical purposes. Still, I can't help but think that people using ozonated swimming pools and spas are absorbing some amount of beneficial oxygen, and no toxic chlorine residues. Medizone also plans an ongoing series of seminars on ozone therapy for the medical community, and the establishment of clinics.

TREATMENT OF HUMAN & PET DISEASE, AGRICULTURE, AND BLOOD BANKS

As we already stated, the patent covers "The inactivation of lipid envelope viruses in blood and blood products normally returned to a mammalian host".

"Lipid envelope viruses" include AIDS, herpes, hepatitis, Epstein-Barr/cytomegalovirus and other viruses. The "mammalian host" as mentioned in the patent, includes: you (people), beef, dairy cattle, chickens, turkeys, hogs, etc., etc.

122

The use of Medizone in agriculture will help eliminate most feedlot disease, and also result in increased herd yields, milk output, and egg production, due to increased cellular efficiencies.

Further, Medizone believes that it's process will also be the end of "incurable" pet diseases like heartworm and cat flu. More proof of the effect of Medizone on disease can be found in the three important scholarly works that Medizone supplied me with as references:

"Ozone Vs. Hepatitis and Herpes - The Choice" by Heinz Konrad, M.D. Brazil.
"Rationale For Treatment of Cancer With Ozone" by Boguslaw Lipinski, Ph.D., Boston.
"Ozone Peroxides - Peroxide Radicals- Oxygen Radicals: What the Ozone Therapist Has To Know About Them" by Dr. R. Viebahn of West Germany, one of the premier ozone researchers of this century.

BLOOD BANKS

Medizone has proven it inactivates viruses inside and outside the body - as in the case of AIDS patients and even blood banks! This will be a godsend to people, like one of my relatives, who got Hepatitis from a blood transfusion during her bypass operation.

When these Medizone treatments are fully implemented, tragedies like this will be a thing of the past, because *all existing blood banks will be able to purify their stored blood supplies by ozonation. It works inside and outside of the body in humans and in animals!* We are truly at the threshold of a new era in health care.

OZONE TV. SPECIAL BEING PRODUCED

The future is so bright for medical ozone, that Threshold Films in Canada has been in touch with Medizone recently. Threshold has spent the past 2 years producing a 60 minute documentary on medical ozone under the auspices of the Canadian Film Board for the CBC, Canadian Television. It features Medizone, and should be finished late in 1988. Threshold Films, #3-OT, 706 W 17th. Ave. Vancouver, B.C. Canada, V5Z IT9, Geoff Rogers, Director and Executive Producer, along with Ryner Derdau, Associate Producer, 604/876-2988.

ONGOING MEDIZONE CLINICAL TRIALS

Medizone has completed one rabbit study, in which, as suspected, the researchers were unable to show any harm or toxicity to the animal by the use of Medizone. It's all up to the FDA, but by late 1988, all the animal toxicity studies should be finished. They have progressed to the feline infectious lukemia studies at Cornell University, toxicity studies using pigs at Mt. Sinai, and wound healing studies. They are advancing successfully on many fronts, and by all rights, will get FDA human testing approval soon.

123

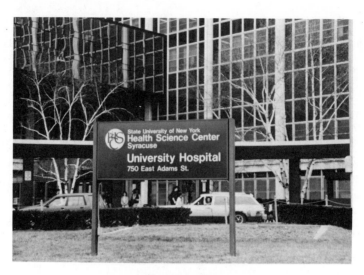

**SYRACUSE UNIVERSITY
SITE OF MEDIZONE LAB STUDIES**

PROOF OF AIDS KILL WITH NO CELL TOXICITY

SYRACUSE NY UNIVERSITY HOSPITAL

At the Syracuse, NY, University Hospital Research Facilities, Dr. Bernard Poiesz has proven that the proper amounts of ozone administered correctly, have achieved a 100% kill ratio of AIDS viruses, both within and outside of the cells, without harming any normal cells! This with no damage to the lymphocytes. More than 10 replications (repeated - for accuracy - tests of the same study) have been completed. The researchers used a hollow fiber bundle process (similar to blood dialysis) to interface ozone with contaminated blood. They used various concentrations, usually around 25 micrograms per cc.

NOTE: Dr. Hugo Veitz (MD) at the Clymer Clinic in Pennsylvania, did ozone work before it was temporarily outlawed in this country. He said he prefers ozone over H_2O_2 because of it's broader flexibility. "You can give practically as little as you want, or go all the way up to 9 or 10 *thousand* micrograms per treatment. Of course, the higher dosages were only given for serious infectious diseases ...in most of the cases you used the lower dosages."

Dr. Poiesz's virology work will interface with Dr. Greenberg's work, at Mt. Sinai, on whole blood effects, becoming a co-publication which will be published in a nationally respected research journal.

MOUNT SINAI HOSPITAL - NEW YORK CITY

Medizone's director of research, Dr. Latino, told me that in the Mount Sinai peripheral blood studies, they used concentrations of 71 micrograms per cc. **This was a concentration level 10 times above what Medizone proposes to use on humans. Even at this elevated level, the researchers only ended up with 5 to 6% hemolysis** (cell destruction). Normal blood cells wear out (from battering) at a rate of 3% anyway. So, when the concentrations are brought down to normal, there should only be the normal cell loss, which is being replaced by the bone marrow. Even at these levels, the extra 3% or so were probably weak. Dr. Latino further stated that, in most studies, anything up to 15% is considered acceptable.

Wound healing studies were also done at Mt. Sinai, and the only problems there were mechanical, where the diminished state animals accidentally breathed the ozone gas being applied to their external wounds. Any rats treated correctly recovered.

LONG ISLAND COLLEGE OF PHARMACY

Other rabbit non-toxicity studies, where blood was drawn out of the animals, ozonated, and reintroduced to the animal, were performed at the Long Island University School of Pharmacy. The results should be published in the medical journals soon. The only thing at all toxic was a slight rise in the uric acid levels. Such an occurrence would only bother someone with gout. In this case, as well, the concentrations were artificially high, and it is suspected that at the proper levels, there will be no problem.

MEDIZONE'S BLUE RIBBON MEDICAL RESEARCHERS

Overseeing the lab studies is a top notch medical board: Jeffrey S. Freed, MD, FACS Assistant Clinical Professor, Mt. Sinai School of Medicine, Joseph S. Latino, Ph.D., Director of Hematology and Oncology Laboratories, Brooklyn Hospital, Glenn Hammer, MD, Assistant Clinical Professor of Medicine, Mt. Sinai, Hubert Weinberg, MD, Assistant Professor, Mt. Sinai School of Medicine, and George White, Ph.D. By the way, Dr. Latino, the director of research, has emphasized that "ozone is blatantly non-toxic".

LENGTH OF TESTS

By law, the FDA human testing procedure has three phases, each may take three months. Medizone anticipates that once their research protocol is approved by the FDA, the phase 1 "clinical trial" will take 12 weeks. This is the trial which determines that there is no (or an acceptable level of) toxicity in humans.

Phase 2 and 3 of the studies, once approved, will consist of human tests anticipated to each take 3 months, plus time between them for FDA review. This whole human test process should take 1 year.

PLEASE RESTRAIN YOURSELF

The last thing Medizone needs or wants at this stage is phone calls from people wanting treatment. By law, they have absolutely nothing to offer, in public or private, and such phone calls will only slow them down from getting the groundwork accomplished so the FDA can grant approval. The only place I know of where one may currently get legal ozone therapy is in Mexico or Germany, or on an experimental basis in a VA hospital. If anywhere else is doing it, please write, and let me know.

Note: Anyone taking ozone treatments may want to investigate the use of antioxidant enzymes. See the section on SOD further on in this book.

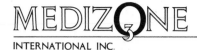

INTERNATIONAL INC.

March 28, 1988

Dear Mr. McCabe,

Since the identification of Acquired Immune Deficiency Syndrome
(AIDS), researchers have employed many modalities to treat
patients with HIV-related disease. In Germany, one modality they
have used is an oxygen/ozone mixture. The mixture was introduced
into fixed volumes of patients' blood _ex vivo_. The procedure was
named autohemotherapy. Anecdotal reports on the results of that
work were extremely encouraging. However, in view of the fact
that no controlled trials were performed, these results must be
carefully evaluated.

In March, 1986, Medizone International, Inc. was created
specifically to scientifically evaluate this treatment. A series
of studies were undertaken to establish:

a)   the safety of autohemotherapy with an
      ozone/oxygen (Medizone) mixture in an animal
      model (toxicity studies);

b)   the effect(s) of ozone/oxygen mixture
      (Medizone) on human target cell line, HUT-78
      (toxicity studies);

c)   the anti-retroviral activity of oxygen/ozone
      (Medizone) on HIV _in vitro_;

d)   the effect of ozone/oxygen (Medizone) in
      human peripheral blood _ex vivo_.

The studies and results to date include:

a)   An animal model treated with (ozone/oxygen)
      Medizone in a manner analogous to the
      proposed human treatment regime at the Long
      Island College of Pharmacy revealed no
      toxicity at concentrations up to ten times
      the dose proposed in man. This study is now
      being repeated to verify the data.

b)   Cell-free HIV treated with (ozone/oxygen)
      Medizone resulted in a 75% inactivation of
      the virus with a single pulse of the drug

that maintains total HUT-78 viability. More recently, a 96% reduction in viral expression has been detected in an ozone flow chamber. These studies were performed at Syracuse University under the auspices of Dr. Bernard Poiesz.

c) Treatment of human peripheral blood with Medizone revealed hemolysis and coagulation changes well within the standard for re-infusion of packed human blood. This study was performed at the Mount Sinai School of Medicine in New York, under the auspices of Dr. Michael Greenberg.

The hypotheses underlying ozone's virucidal activity are based upon the drug's propensity toward lipid peroxidation. Those viruses which are lipid-encapsulated (i.e. lentivirus family) are highly susceptible to the direct oxidative effect of ozone, and are thereby inactivated. Data (both referenced and submitted), indicate the differential effect on lipid-envelope viruses versus those whose lipid capsid composition is minimal.

We postulate that ozone will inactivate cell-incorporated viruses by two mechanisms:

1) Due to the high degree of lipid peroxidation catalyzed by ozone interaction(s), viral binding to specific receptors (i.e. HIV to CD_{4A} receptor), whose membraneous nature implies a finite composition of lipid [including polyunsaturated fatty acids (PUFA)], may indeed be ozone sensitive. Investigations with Rhodamine-labelled HIV, exposed to target cells pre-sensitized with ozone, may suggest alterations in receptor/ligand binding capacity yielding diminished viral binding.

2) It has been demonstrated that target cells with pro-viral DNA incorporated into its genome have decreased titers of certain protective enzyme systems with respect to oxidative perturbations. In particular, superoxide dismutase (SOD), catalase (CAT) and glutathione peroxidase (GSHPx) levels are diminished in a number of virally transformed cell lines. Such decreases may render oxidative effects initiated by ozone. It should be noted that ozone's effects are instantaneous with regard to peroxidation and the products of this reaction (hydroperoxides) with cellular membrane lipids are relatively stable and can participate in a host of oxidative (including

free-radical) propagating reactions.

It is our intention to generate, via ozone's reaction with cellular membranes, hydroperoxides measurable by the thiobarbituric acid assay, sufficient to:

a) inactivate cell-free virus (in concert with direct ozone effects);

b) reduce cell incorporation of virus by blocking viral-receptor binding;

c) inactivate cell-incorporated virus in HUT-78 infected cells rendering them non-viable while maintaining normal target cell viability.

The results of experimental work have demonstrated non-toxicity in treating an animal model, human HIV target cells and human peripheral blood with an ozone/oxygen mixture (Medizone). Anti-retroviral activity was demonstrated at concentrations maintaining HUT-78 viability. We have presented sound hypotheses for a non-toxic treatment for AIDS.

During the last eighteen months the results of each of these studies have encouraged Medizone International, Inc. to pursue an IND for human clinical trials for the drug ozone/oxygen (Medizone) in the treatment of HIV infection.

If you have any questions, please do not hesitate to call.

Yours sincerely,

Terrence O. McGrath
Chief Executive Officer

The Biochemical Processes Underlying Ozone Therapy

Ozone has properties with significant medical applications: it is bactericidal, fungicidal, virucidal and enhances circulation.

Virucidal

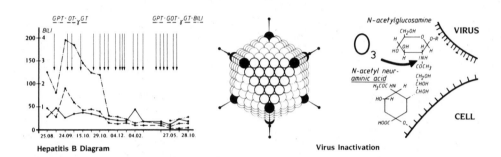

Hepatitis B Diagram

Virus Inactivation

Enhances Circulation

Biochemistry of glycosis influenced by peroxides

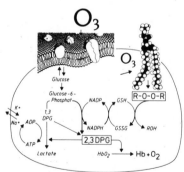

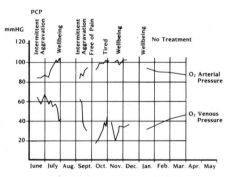

Every increase in 2,3 DPG facilitates the release of oxygen through a shifting of the HbO$_2$/Hb balance in favor of deoxygenated hemoglobin.

It is possible, by measurement of the arterial and venous pressures pO$_2$, to observe in vivo the change in the oxygen situation during the course of treatment.

By Dr. rer. nat. Renate Viebahn
Dr. J. Hansler Gmbh. Nordring 8, D-7551 Iffezheim (W. Germany)

BUCK McCABE

I interviewed Buck McCabe (no relation to myself), and found out some fascinating things that show ozone in a very favorable light. Buck stated that he was once the director of a geothermal power plant that was 43% controlled by Dow Chemical. In this position, he met people knowledgeable about ozone. Soon, he became interested in ozone's medical applications, started researching the field, and after much research, decided to take it up. Being interested, but still skeptical, he went to Europe and systematically arrived unannounced, at the front doors of all the major ozone using MD's. He did this to be sure he got the straight story from each. He visited and studied the treatment facilities of "ozonating" doctors, in Germany, Switzerland, Italy, & Belgium.

Buck found the European doctors typically prudent and reserved, sort of "old world" types who never made any exaggerated claims, yet were producing fascinating results using ozone in the treatment of disease. Buck even made friends with Dr. Renate Viebahn, and studied her methods as well.

He was so impressed with what he saw, that he bought a variety of the most advanced medical ozone machines available: 3 Hansler PM83's, 2 Biozone computer controlled 13T's, a Vacazone, and 3 Vapozone (ozone fog) units. He moved these machines to Mexicali, Baja California, and put together a nonprofit medical civic organization. He created a top notch medical clinic, and staffed it with 3 doctors. In 1985, and even now, his "Clinica Medica De Ozono Therapia" was the largest medical ozone clinic ever in operation. The clinic treated over 4,000 patients!

Earlier in the book, we spoke of the history of ozone usage in Europe. What's the difference between the Europeans and what Buck was doing? In Europe, thousands of doctors have one machine each, and because their medical system doesn't require them to publish papers, there is simply no national database for us to see. They have just been quietly treating people with ozone for over 30 years. Buck McCabe was doing it, "big time", and had more machines in operation in one place, at one time, than anyone ever had before.

Mr. McCabe stated that his clinic achieved an average 70% success rate, "success" as defined by contemporary medicine, for lukemia. In operation for 25 months, the clinic closed down due to the staggering Mexican inflation rate, causing the price of supplies to go up 900%. Treating a patient population of 4,000 probably makes them some of the most experienced clinicians ever.

As far as protocols and dosages go, the clinic usually adjusted them according to the disease being treated and followed the directions supplied by the manufacturers of the individual machines they were using, usually the Hansler & Biozone units. The Vapozone ozone fog generating equipment was inherently a fixed dosage design. The highest concentration ever injected were 108 micro milligrams. That's a very small amount, 180 over a millionth of a gram. The lowest used was 22.

131

Buck's clinic usually started a patient on 22, and judged what the patient could tolerate, raising the concentrations in succeeding sessions to 35 or 40. Buck knows some doctors experimenting with dosages of 60 or 65, amounts that Buck considers to be very high concentrations. His experience showed him that "using a high concentration just doesn't seem to do the job", and "lower ozone concentrations are better". in this case, Buck's experience showed him the best window of effectiveness to be 22 to 40 micro milligrams.

In order of "the most success" listed first, here are all the major diseases they worked with: gangrene usually required a one hour session each day, with ozone being put in the blood, and into a gas bag. However, out of a total of 33 patients scheduled for surgical amputation, only 1 (with other problems, too,) actually had to have an amputation. Arthritis was usually treated every other day, and within 3 days there was significant reduction of pain, and by the end of the patient's stay, deformed joints were reduced as a matter of course. Herpes (all types were affected), Lupus, & Parkinson's disease. The Orthopedic Hospital in Los Angeles would also send him patients to be treated for Muscular Dystrophy.

Buck's clinic also treated many other insurance patients from the U.S., for a whole variety of diseases, on a regular basis. At the time, Buck considered learning how to interface with the U. S. insurance industry as a significant accomplishment. They called the therapy "Chemohemotherapy".

Did he treat AIDS patients? The answer was surprising. Where they were located, in Mexico, there were only 4 AIDS cases in the huge local population. If they had brought AIDS patients in for treatment, they were sure the locals would have burnt down their facility, so they dared not treat AIDS victims.

I asked Buck if he was ever able to publish any results or issue totals of patient records. He said unfortunately, no. They were all so overworked with their clinical duties that they simply didn't have the time.

We also discussed industrial ozone usage here in the U.S., and I was surprised to find out how widespread it's use is: several thousand used car dealers use ozone machines to remove smoke and other odors from cars they clean up for resale, giving them that "fresh" smell. Motels give rooms a 10 minute treatment to freshen them up by sterilization, and Convention centers are using ozone to prevent Legionaire's disease contamination through air systems.

In 1991, Federal law will require municipalities to eliminate chlorine from drinking water supplies. Ozone is the most effective, and least expensive alternative. Los Angeles city drinking water is now ozonated, and they will soon be building other new plants. To show you how quickly this technology is developing, look at the Thomas Register's listings of Ozone companies. 3 years ago, there were only 4. Today there's about 30, and we're just getting started. Japan has become a major manufacturer of ozone units. The surprising thing, is the lack of interest shown by the major U.S. corporations in entering this exploding growth market. With their tremendous resources, we could become the leaders in ozone technology, instead of watching other countries do it.

INDUSTRIAL OZONE

INDUSTRIAL OZONE GENERATION IS BIG BUSINESS

There are million-dollar corporations installing giant ozone generators all over the world. These industrial installations are quietly cleaning up municipal and private water supplies, swimming pools, and industrial contamination sites. For a complete listing, contact IOA and go to the library and look up "Ozone" in the Thomas Register. In this book alone, there are over 30 listed, with big ads and pictures of both enormous and small lab units. Some do over $50 million in sales, per year. Some are electrode produced, some are UV (ultraviolet). Go to a big Pool & Spa show, ozone generator companies will be there too.

Here's a newspaper article:

USE OF OZONE YIELDS DRINKING WATER FREE OF BACTERIA, CHLORINE AFTERTASTE

- HEADLINE: NEWARK STAR-LEDGER SPECIAL REPORT
May 19, 1988 by Gordon Bishop

Ozone - a key ingredient in creating suffocating smog, as well as a life-protecting shield against deadly radiation is now being hailed as the best way of attacking bacteria in drinking water supplies. Ozone, a form of oxygen, can either harm or improve life on Earth, depending on how it's used. As a substitute for chlorine, ozone can kill bacteria without the side effects caused by chlorine, including possible cancerous diseases and hardening of the arteries.

About 30 of the nation's 60,000 water companies, including the Hackensack, New Jersey, Water Co., have turned to ozone to destroy bacteria and viruses in their water treatment plants. Unlike chlorine, a deadly gas, ozone does not spin off such cancer-causing "precursors" as trihalomethanes or chloroform. In water, ozone (after it does its job on the agents of infectious diseases) changes back to normal, life-sustaining oxygen, within 30 minutes. For that chemically miraculous reason, Hackensack Water will be treating its drinkable supplies with ozone by next year. "Consumers will notice obvious improvements at the tap," said Thomas McKeon, vice president of operations at Hackensack Water, the state's largest purveyor, with nearly a million consumers. "Ozone is an effective bactericide and inactivates viruses better than chlorine" And it's cheaper, too, in the overall treatment process. The company expects to save $10 Million in construction costs. An additional savings of $25 million will be realized in operations over the life of the $65 million, $220-million gallon-per-day treatment plant. The facility will be the second largest in the U.S.

133

INDUSTRIAL OZONE GENERATORS

Randomly picked companies from the Thomas Register:

Water Management Inc. P.O. Box 2552-OT, Escondido, CA, 92025. Manufacture their own lamps in Holland, world wide installers of large turnkey systems. These are the PHOTOZONE PROCESS people I feature in the section after this one.

BHK 1000-OT S. Magnolia Ave. Monrovia, CA. (818)357-9667. UV Sources - mercury lamps

Voltarc Tubes Dept. A-OT, P.O.B. 688 Fairfield, CT 06430 203/255-2633 Ozone generating & specialty lamps

Air Neutralizer Corp. 1600-OT VFW Parkway, W. Roxbury, MA

Ozone Research & Equipment Corp. 3840 North 40th Ave. Dept. OT, Phoenix, AZ 85019-3613, 602/272-2681 Ozone monitors, large and small.

Ozone Technology Inc. 2113 Anthony Drive Dept. OT, Tyler TX, 75703 214/581-2060 Ozone treatment of bacteria & viruses.

Infilco Degremont, Inc. P.O.B. 29599 Dept. M-OT, Richmond, VA 23229 800/4461150 804/281-7600 Large systems 50lbs./day. They were nice enough to supply the photos of the industrial units in this book.

Howe Baker Engineers, Process Systems International, P.O.B. 956-OT Tyler, TX 75710 214/561-5551 "Sonozaire" Odor Neutralizer

PCI Ozone Corporation, One-OT Fairfield Crescent, West Caldwell, NJ 07006 American Ultraviolet Co Dept OT, 32 Commerce Street, Chatham, NJ

Atlantic Ultraviolet Corp. Dept OT, 250 North Fehr Way, Bay Shore, NY 11706 516/586-5900 - Nice people, I met Ann Wysocki, Comptroler, at an Agricultural trade show where they were selling units to ozonate/purify water for farm stock animals. Their list of installations looks like a "Who's Who" of corporate America.

MEDICAL OZONE GENERATORS

Biozon Ozon-Technik GmbH, An Der Haune #10, Bad Hersfeld, D-6430, Federal Republic of Germany, manufactures ozone generators for medical use.

Hansler Ozone units from Germany will probably be sold by Medizone.

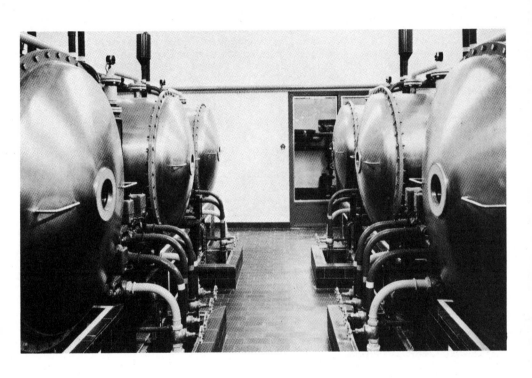

**INDUSTRIAL OZONE GENERATORS
COURTESY INFILCO DEGREMONT INC.**

THE INTERNATIONAL OZONE ASSN. IOA

Headquartered in Zurich, Switzerland, The International Ozone Association (IOA) has an office in Norwalk, CT. A membership organization open to professionals and the public, they supply their members "Ozone Science and Engineering" and "Ozone News".

IOA holds regular U.S. professional conferences and courses on such subjects as "Ozonation Systems: Design, Operation and Maintenance", targeted for managers and operators of "ozonation facilities, water and wastewater treatment plants, and water supplies, especially appropriate in view of the 1986 Amendments to the U.S. Safe Drinking Water Act (proposed regulations on Surface Water Treatment and Total Coliform).

IOA PUBLICATIONS:
Who's Who In Ozone
Ozonation Manual For Water and Wastewater Treatment - 1982
Proceedings of Ozone World Congress
Applications of Ozone in Water Treatment
Ozonation - Environmental Impact and Benefit
Ozone and Biology
International Ozone Symposium - Wasser Berlin 1985
Ozone and Ultra-Violet Water Treatment
Analytical Aspects of Ozone Ground Water Quality Protection
Rural Ground Water Contamination
Toxic Contamination In Large Lakes
Aquatic Applications of Ozone
Forum on Ozone Disinfection
Design and Operation of Ozone Systems for Drinking Water Plants

IOA Pan American Committee, 83-OT Oakwood Avenue, Norwalk, CT 06850

OZONE LAMP SOURCES

Commercial ozone trace emission spectra producing lamps can be purchased through General Electric, Westinghouse-Phillips, (look for both in the phone book). Also, from Voltarc - 176-OT Linwood Avenue, Fairfield Ct. 06430-0688, (203) 2552633

The special concentrated Photozone lamps (available in large quantities only) from: Water Management, Inc. (see Photozone section below)

Also check the Thomas Register at your library, and local swimming pool and spa suppliers and stores. Pet stores sell tank ozonators.

POOLS AND SPAS

DEL INDUSTRIES

"Researchers are finding that water in public aquatic facilities may be more contaminated than raw sewage treatment plants" - Golf Course Management, April 1986. Home pool, and spa, ozonation is quite widespread, having been in use for 50 years. If you swim in ozonated water, I imagine you must get some oxygen into your system through the skin. Depending on the concentration, the odor ranges from slightly sweet, to moderately antiseptic. Del Industries is one of the leaders in this market, "The nation's #1 selling ozone generator for spas." They use the trade name "Delzone."

Their products: Delzone - ozone generator used for up to 1,200 gallons, Delpak - complete automatic ozone package for spas, Del Ozone Sweep - automatic pool cleaner and ozonator, Del Poolzone - pools up to 90,000 gallons, Del Poolpak - automatic ozone package for aboveground pools, Delflo - Ozone dispersion system, Del Switch - automatic pressure switch, plus check valves and timers. They also offer Del Pure, "The only complete home water treatment system that works naturally - chemical free.

The ultraviolet bulbs in Del spa units last about 7,500 hours, and in Del pool units 12,000 hours. They use about 25 watts. If you run the units 24 hours a day, you'll just waste energy, and any ozone not used for purification will convert back to oxygen. Ultraviolet sterilizers are not the same, as they only treat the water that passes by them, not the whole pool.

OZONE LASTS LONGER THAN USUALLY THOUGHT

Conventional wisdom states that ozone disappears after 20-30 minutes, but Wayne R. Hruden has published: "Preliminary Investigations of Ozone in Recreational Water - Jan 87," in which he reports detection of ozone levels in water, after 12 hours.

Del Industries 223-OT Granada Drive, San Luis Obispo, CA 93401

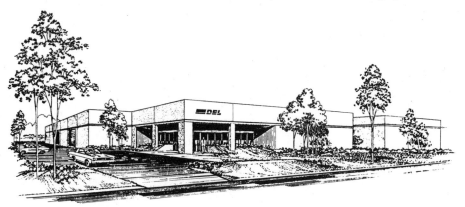

SPA PRODUCTS

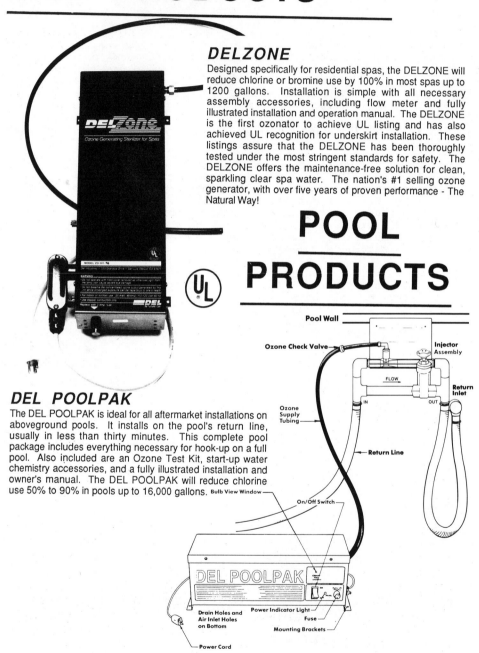

DELZONE

Designed specifically for residential spas, the DELZONE will reduce chlorine or bromine use by 100% in most spas up to 1200 gallons. Installation is simple with all necessary assembly accessories, including flow meter and fully illustrated installation and operation manual. The DELZONE is the first ozonator to achieve UL listing and has also achieved UL recognition for underskirt installation. These listings assure that the DELZONE has been thoroughly tested under the most stringent standards for safety. The DELZONE offers the maintenance-free solution for clean, sparkling clear spa water. The nation's #1 selling ozone generator, with over five years of proven performance - The Natural Way!

POOL
PRODUCTS

DEL POOLPAK

The DEL POOLPAK is ideal for all aftermarket installations on aboveground pools. It installs on the pool's return line, usually in less than thirty minutes. This complete pool package includes everything necessary for hook-up on a full pool. Also included are an Ozone Test Kit, start-up water chemistry accessories, and a fully illustrated installation and owner's manual. The DEL POOLPAK will reduce chlorine use 50% to 90% in pools up to 16,000 gallons.

Pool Wall

Ozone Check Valve

Injector Assembly

FLOW

Return Inlet

Ozone Supply Tubing

IN   OUT

Return Line

Bulb View Window

On/Off Switch

DEL POOLPAK

Drain Holes and
Air Inlet Holes
on Bottom

Power Indicator Light

Fuse

Mounting Brackets

Power Cord

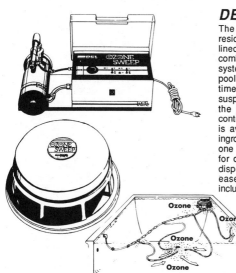

DEL OZONE SWEEP

The DEL OZONE SWEEP is designed for any shape residential pool, inground or aboveground, including vinyl-lined pools, up to 30,000 gallons. The ozone generator combines with a dispersion pump and a unique, patented system which disperses ozone evenly throughout the whole pool, eliminating chlorine use 90% to 100%. At the same time, four cleaning whips agitate particulate dirt into suspension for removal by the filter, automatically cleaning the pool. The DEL OZONE SWEEP features a master control panel for easy operation. The DEL OZONE SWEEP is available in three models. There are two models for inground pools: 110 volt with a built-in GFI, and 220 volt, and one 110 volt aboveground pool model which features a timer for overall filter system control and has the ozonator and dispersion pump assembled and mounted on a base for ease of installation. Everything needed for installation, including a fully illustrated manual, is included.

HOUSEHOLD WATER PURIFICATION

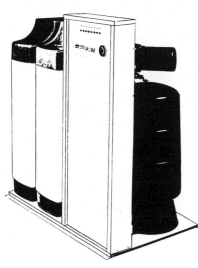

DELPURE

DEL's latest addition to our comprehensive line of Ozone purification systems is the DELPURE. It is the only complete home water treatment system that works naturally - chemical-free! The DELPURE purifies all of the water coming into the home and removes contaminants such as iron, heavy metals, cyanide, arsenic, etc. All the water is filtered and sterilized. The DELPURE will enhance and improve taste, smell, and clarity of the water. Now all household water will be as fresh as bottled water for just pennies per day.

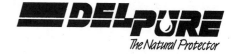

The Natural Protector

THE PHOTOZONE PROCESS

The developer of the Photozone Advanced Photo Oxidation Ozone process is Mr. Andrew Pincon, President of Water Management Inc., (WMI). WMI's ozone system installation corporation has expanded rapidly and now includes two offices in the United States, with subsidiary offices in Norway, Holland, and Singapore. Water Management Inc. is a consulting engineering firm that designs, builds, and installs "turnkey" ozone system installations. Their prices range from $5 thousand, to $5 million dollars in cost. At present, they have over 4,000 systems installed worldwide. Mr. Pincon states that he was the original advocate of U.S. swimming pool and spa ozonation starting back in 1974.

TRADITIONAL TECHNOLOGY

In the usual classical ozone generation technology, an ozone generator has 8,000 to 20,000 volts of electricity inside it. Incoming dehumidified and cooled room air passes over the generator's charged electrodes, producing ozone. In this method, everything in the air (including any water or nitrogen) is heated and indiscriminately ionized.

Our normal air contains 20% oxygen and 79% nitrogen. The nitrogen in the air ionizes quickly. If you will remember this book's section on "cold process" ozone we saw how corrosive nitric acid is usually formed as a by-product of classic "hot spark" ozone generation. Photozone does not have this drawback. There are certain high frequency "corona brush" ozone production units that are also supposedly acid free, the "Octazone" method out of Germany is one such example.

NEW TECHNOLOGY

As we have seen in the previous section about the lab researcher, "Cold process" or "nitric oxide free" types of ozone can be formed from special "ceramic sandwich" composition generators. Cold process ozone can also be formed from air or water that is subjected to high frequencies or ultraviolet light. The amount and type of ozone produced depends on the wavelength of the light being used. The closer we come to the natural sun produced ozone, the less problems there are.

Scientists consider light to be a stream of invisible packets or compressions of energy that are called photons or waves. The energy carried by a light's photons increases as the length of the light's wave (wavelength) shortens. Only the UV light that is actually absorbed causes any chemical or physical changes, and atoms and molecules absorb only those wavelengths that provide the right frequency of energy to produce any changes to their state.

Let's examine the differences between the traditional commercially produced ozone and the special UV lamp Photozone gas:

PHOTOZONE AND TRADITIONAL HOT SPARK OZONE COMPARED

Photozone	*Ozone*
Negative Ions	Positive Ions
pH Basic	pH Acid
No nitrogen oxides	Nitrogen oxides present
2+ hour half-life in tap water	20 minute half-life in tap water
66% negatively charged ozone	96.4% positively charged ozone

As you can see from the above comparison chart, the patented Photozone Advanced Photo Oxidation (APO) process, generates ozone, but has some significant differences: The special Photozone UV lamps produce the exact wavelengths needed to produce not only ozone, but other higher forms of activated oxygen as well. No significant corrosive nitric oxides are present. The gas is full of negative ions. Note the similarity to the negative ion avalanche effect noted by the Japanese physicist in the section on cold process ozone. An analysis of the compounds in Photozone gas are as follows:

COMPOUNDS IN PHOTOZONE ACTIVATED OXYGEN GAS

Ozone, O_3, 66.7%
Hydroxy Radical, OH, 14.7%
Hydroperoxy Radical, HO_2, 6.3%
Hydrogen Peroxide, H_2O_2, 5.9%
Atomic Oxygen, O, 4.4%
Other Oxidants, 2.0%
Nitrogen Oxides, NO, <0.1%

NOTE: Please notice the presence of our friends, the peroxide radicals, and hydrogen peroxide. You will find them explained in detail in the previous sections on medical uses of ozone, and hydrogen peroxide.

SPECIAL UV LAMPS

For the answer on how WMI produces these special Photozone ozone compounds, we quote Mr. Pincon, again, who states: "We produce oxidants photochemically in the vacuum ultraviolet range by manufacturing our own lamps in our factory in Holland. Our lamps give off light in wavelengths of 150 to 200 nanometers. Most UV/ozone suppliers are assemblers, using lamps from G.E. & Westinghouse (now Phillips), who's mercury vapor lamps usually give an average emission spectra line of 254 nanometers, and less than 1% of it is at 185nm, which is a trace kind of spectra. Consequently, the concentration of gases from mercury lamps is usually not of an industrial amount, and they are used primarily in spas and swimming pools or hospitals for sterilization."

The Photozone lamps emit much shorter wavelengths, which produce photons with a higher than usual energy. This higher energy charge creates, not only "cold process" ozone, but other highly active oxygen compounds usually not found in traditional

141

ozone generation. Most importantly, less than .1% nitrogen oxides
are created. In other words, toxic by-products are not formed, as
in classical ozone generation. The proprietary Photozone activated
oxygen generation produces "aprocess ozone" O_3-, by using duterium
and xenon gas lamps, with light emission frequencies much lower
than 185nm.

AVAILABILITY AND USEFUL LIFE OF SPECIAL OZONE PRODUCING LAMPS

At this time, Water Management Inc. only sells total
generating systems, not just the lamps, "unless someone wants a
thousand of them." The smallest unit they sell is about 20" long
and around 40 watts, but it handles well in excess of 80,000
gallons of water per day. By their third year of continuous use, a
Photozone lamp only looses 10 to 15% of it's output, having over 5
times the output of a normal 36" lamp. The people at WMI consider
themselves supplying the state-of-the-art in ozone production
technology.

A STEP ELIMINATED

This technology is a breakthrough in simplicity. Usually we
filter contaminants out of water, not by destroying them, but by
removing them and putting them someplace else. You filter out the
toxins, the filter is filled up, and you still have toxic waste,
but now it's in a filter that still needs to be put somewhere,
where it won't harm anything. The beauty of an ozone process is
the elimination of this extra step, by immediate oxidation of the
contaminants into harmless by-products:

END PRODUCTS OF CONTAMINANTS TREATED WITH PHOTOZONE

Carbon Dioxide
Water
Oxygen
Filterable Solids
Dissolved Halides (such as chlorine & bromide)

BENEFITS OF AN OZONE WITHOUT TOXIC CONTAMINANTS

Without the interference of unwanted thermally bonded nitrogen
oxides, the activated oxygen compounds work much more efficiently.
Plus, the incoming air doesn't need to be dehumidified since the
nitrogen in the air passes through without combining with airborne
humidity along the way. Photozone ozone and it's extra forms of
active oxygen react with any pollutants or microbes, just as
traditional ozone does, and have the added benefit of being
economical enough to use in large commercial applications as well.
Even though it is less expensive to produce, the Photozone gas has
26% more oxidizing power than conventionally generated ozone, and
91% more oxidizing power than chlorine!

USES OF ACTIVATED OXYGEN

The Photozone treated process water is used to remove biological and chemical contamination. Bacteria, algae, fungi, cyst and virus metabolisms are ruptured during biological chemical oxidation. Destruction of algae and cysts can also occur through chemical oxidation of their cell walls. Detoxification of bad-smelling hazardous sewage and hazardous chemical pollution occurs because the Photozone gas "cleaves" their chemical bonds" and ruptures the molecular structure of the toxic substances into lighter weight non-toxic molecular fragments. It is efficient in destroying the following microorganisms: E. Coli, Staphylococcus aureus, Pseudomonas aeruginosa, and Proteus mirabilis.

The Activated Oxygen produced by the Photozone process has been used in a variety of chemical treatment processes, including oxidation of heavy metals, taste and odor compounds, color, phenols, and volatile organic compounds.

CURRENT POLLUTION CLEANUP USES OF ACTIVATED OXYGEN

Our society has an overabundance of pollution and disease problems begging for solutions. Many solutions already exist, but you simply have never heard of them, and neither have our municipal engineers. Here's a few examples of applications already in use.

The increasing pollution of our oceans has seriously damaged our ocean-based food sources. An example is oysters. The state of Texas recently prohibited further sale of local oysters unless they were first transferred to clean breeding grounds, or purified somehow. In New Orleans, WMI has the only permit in the United States, allowing the taking of a shellfish harvest from shellfish grounds closed because of microbiological toxic contamination. Here's why: First, they collect and transport each inedible toxic oyster harvest directly to their labs. Then, a crew, including 3 full time microbiologists, places the oysters in tanks filled with circulating Photozone process water. The oysters in the tank draw in and expell the Photozone treated water and purify themselves! The once toxic oysters are now safe for human consumption.

The Photozone process has cleaned up salmon hatcheries, restored duck ponds, restored lakes up to 300 acres, cleaned dolphin pools, controlled red tide, cleaned shark tanks, and disinfected seawater. Because both fish gills and Photozone gas carry negative electric charges, they are not attracted to each other and the fish suffer no discomfort. In fish hatcheries, Photozone kills bacteria and parasites, removes the fish waste nitrogen compounds (by converting nitrites to nitrates), and aerates the water with fresh oxygen. Heavy industry applications? No problem. JPL (Jet Propulsion Laboratories) polluted the groundwater at Pasadena, where their processes discharged a number of contaminants into the ground. Now they use APO to clean up their aquifer. Water Management Inc. also does other hazardous waste site leeching cleanup, eliminating benzine, trithalomethanes, pesticides, complex cyanide, phenols, TCE, PCE, EDB, and PCB's, etc.

143

SPORTS AND RECREATION

While we're at it let's examine sports and recreation. In another case, WMI installed their Photozone process in the Los Angeles pools used for the 1984-85 Olympic Games. Several Olympic competitors and coaches remarked about the clarity of water and how the pool did not feel as though it had been chemically treated. The Photozone ozone system is still in place, and the buildup of scum, algae and corrosive chlorine odors has virtually been eliminated in an indoor pool at the same site. Today the coaches say the athletes take the water out of the one million six hundred thousand gallon pool & bring it home to drink. They believe it's more beneficial, and tastes better than their L.A. city tap water! In fact, WMI claims it can give your pool a degree of purity equal to that required in hospital therapy pools, at less cost then you are paying now.

ECONOMIC SAVINGS OF OZONE

Look at these typical economics: The hydrotherapy pool at Penrose hospital in Colorado Springs, Colorado, put in a Photozone unit. They previously had to empty and clean the pool every one to four weeks. Now the pool has been drained only twice in 21 months of operation without any loss of water quality. This has saved about 281,000 gallons of water, $4,536, and resulted in a system payback time of only 12 months! And that's even before taking into consideration the reduced maintenance labor for filling chemical feeders, scrubbing the pool, etc.

A shrimp hatchery installed a Photozone treatment process and production increased from 3 million postlarvae to over 18 million postlarvae per month! The shrimp survival rate then increased from 20% to over 80%! Tinker Air Force Base in Oklahoma City has the largest electroplating facilities in the world. They provide all the electroplating services for the Army, Air Force and Marine Corps. Because of this they also have a big toxic waste problem. Their chemical processes produced Cyanide and other toxins that were discharged into the local environment as waste products. Now they use the Photozone activated oxygen process, at 400 gallons per minute, to detoxify their ground water. At a considerable savings, they have solved their cyanide toxic waste problem.

Ozone drinking water supply purification has been accomplished at many commercial resorts. In one recent resort installation, WMI came in at an overall cost of only $0.08 per 1,000 gallons treated, 30% less than the conventional alternative.

MOST U.S. MUNICIPALITIES UNAWARE OF PROCESS

If you are one of the few people who has never heard of Giardiasis, consider yourself lucky. Municipal water supplies throughout the country are threatened by this parasite. If you drink Giardia parasites in your tap water, they cause severe and persistent diarrhea, and are untreatable by normal purification methods. Giardia lamblia is the most common waterborne disease in this country, and the most common threat to our drinking water today. Luckily, the Photozone process can not only remove, but kill Giardia at half the cost of other alternatives. Upon contact

144

with the activated oxygen gas, they shrivel up and die. Reminds you of oxygenation products attacking viruses and toxins in the body, doesn't it? Upcoming federal drinking water quality requirements are becoming increasingly stringent, and water utilities nationwide will have to reevaluate the adequacy of existing and proposed water treatment facilities.

Ozone water treatment has a long history of proven, tested, safe, efficient use. The reason ozone is not being used enough in this country is a marketing problem, not a scientific one. Ozone has been purifying water in the U.S. and Europe since the early 1900's. Currently there are over 1,000 active drinking water treatment plants using ozone to make water clear again, remove organic solids, disinfect it, decontaminate it, and solve taste and odor problems. Even though this technology exists, it is not presently used in the U.S. nearly as often as it should be. Most decision makers, and especially the public, are unaware of it's existence. If someone has heard of it, they usually only know of the old (more expensive and more maintenance intensive) processes, and are unaware of the new technologies offering lower costs and maintenance expenses.

Many cities have incorrectly assumed that bad tasting, questionable water is a fact of modern life. Europeans, however, demand and receive ozone purified municipal water. They simply will not put up with the taste of chlorine. In the U.S., I don't see where the public even knows it has a choice. One of the further reasons I wrote this book, "Oxygen Therapies".

NEW COST EFFICIENCIES

The Photozone process presents a major breakthrough in the cost of ozone. Because there are no nitrogen compounds like nitric acid formed, any project using ozone won't have it's plant equipment subject to the same corrosion as in a traditional ozone system. Also, because the incoming air source does not need drying and cooling prior to it's treatment, there is no large expenditure or maintenance for dehumidification and air conditioning. It would be nice to see the day when all municipal water supplies are ozone purified, and producing healthy, pleasant tasting water. Perhaps you could help make this happen.

Water Management Inc./Photozone, may be contacted at P.O. Box 2552-OT, Escondido, CA, and their high-tech, aquaculture shellfish detoxification operation is located in Metairie, Louisiana.

Since we brought up ozone used in the breeding of marine life, I might as well tell a couple of stories to illustrate the widespread disinformation surrounding the subject. "Aquarium buffs" are also involved in our controversies as well. Some claim they have beautiful fish, and clear tanks, because they put ozone in the water, much like our previously mentioned olympic swimming pools.

A new mall opened up nearby, and I wandered into the pet store to see if they sold ozonators, and to find out how the store manager stood on the subject of ozone. He said, "Ozone isn't good for fish," I asked him why, and he showed me, in a resource book, where an "expert" had written that ozone was believed harmful to fish. The author stated that ozone reacted with salts and produced toxins. The author obviously didn't know about the wonderful things being done in breeding tanks by the (previously discussed) Photozone people. She also apparently is unaware that Disney World's, "Living Seas" 6 million gallon tank, Sea World's, "Shark Encounters" and whale tanks, and, The Baltimore Aquarium's fish tanks, are all cleaned by ozone. Also, a German aquarium supply house, Sander, sells aquarium ozonators.

The manager and I got to talking about oxygen and life, and he confided to me that there <u>was</u> a man, in a nearby town, who swore by his fish tank ozonator. He then took me into the back room, and showed me how they kept their display tanks clean. You guessed it, an oxygenator. They had a homemade-type unit that was very similar to the Pendell Water Oxygenator (mentioned later), except, it didn't use pressurized oxygen.

It had what looked like an upside down, rotating lawn sprinkler, positioned just above what looked like a small roll of plastic fence standing on it's edges. The roll of "fence" had spacious styrofoam padding rolled inside each rotation. All of this was in a clear plastic box. The dirty fish tank water came out of the sprinkler head, and was sprayed on top of this roll, and the water ran down over the surfaces. The surface area that the water was exposed to was, thereby, quite large. He explained this was called an "artificial reef", and aerobic bacteria lived on the roll, while digesting any toxins, and purified the water, which was returned to the tank. I noted, that the water was thinned out, as it sprayed over the roll, to the point that it was able to bubble and absorb lots of oxygen. Just like nature's waterfalls.

On another front, I also dropped in on an aquaculture (fish breeding) seminar held at the local college, and asked the lecturer if he ever heard of using ozone to clean his water. He had just complained of the hassles of constantly getting permits, and draining his ponds, cleaning them, and hauling away the waste. His response was, "Ozone is only used to oxygenate tall tanks, not for detoxification." Now here's the interesting part, a few slides later, he showed everyone his fish farm's "Ultraviolet Light Sterilizer." He hadn't realized the connection in his mind, yet, that the UV light sterilized by producing ozone. After he realizes that, he will have to learn how the ozone people use more powerful lamps, and oxidize all the toxins. We see again, how it's a communication and marketing problem, not a technical one.

PILLS, PRODUCTS, PLACES, PROPOSALS, & PATHS

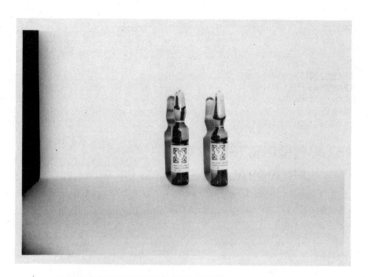

**AMPULES REPORTED TO BE A KOCH TYPE FORMULATION
UNKNOWN COMPOSITION**

DR. WILLIAM F. KOCH, M.D., Ph.D.

Doctor Koch, as a young man, studied under Professor Moses Gomberg. This was extremely beneficial to the young Dr. Koch, because Professor Gomberg, in 1910, discovered the nature of the free radical that we hear so much about today. Dr. Koch earned his doctorate in chemistry as a "free radical specialist", and became a medical doctor, ending up Professor of Chemistry and Histology at the University of Michigan Medical School, and Professor of Physiology at Wayne State University. He came from a family of merit. For example, his uncle, Robert Koch, was a Nobel Laureate who discovered the tuberculosis germ. The head of Dow Chemical Laboratories, Dr. W. Dow, called Dr. William Koch "*The greatest living doctor, a modern Pasteur*", and, Dr. Koch was also praised by Dr. A.R. Mitchell, once the Chairman, Board of Trustees, AMA.

INVENTS POWERFUL OXYGENATORS

Koch produced 1:4 Benzoquinone or Parabenzoquinone in a 1×10^{14} dilution, a catalyst of GLYOXYLIDE (C=O=O=C), that contains the antibiotic radical, and contains it twice, without any inhibitory radical. It is the most unsaturated receptor known.

Note: There is reported to be much more to preparing the formula than just mixing chemicals.

In the 1950's, Koch, and many other doctors and patients, reported that: by using this dilute catalyst, he was able to rid people of diabetes, lukemia, cancer, leprosy, allergy and tuberculosis. A catalyst is something that causes a reaction, but doesn't enter into it. Like a match starts a forest fire which keeps on burning without the match. He said that his catalyst "Restored the oxidation mechanism of waste products of the body, by use of an oxidation starter". He further stated that, **toxins** (waste products of incomplete metabolism) **accumulate in the system because sickness or injury slows or stops the normal immune system function of digesting them.** Not being oxidized, these waste products pile up in the cells. This is called lowered metabolism and often results in cancer and other disease. Where cancer appears to result from injury or irritation, the real cause is toxic build up at the site. **His catalyst took toxins piled up in the body, and converted them into antitoxins. These new antitoxins would then convert other toxins into antitoxins, and the cycle repeated itself over and over. The reaction would continue on for months, cleaning out the body.**

He was sued by the FDA. Because the formula was in parts per trillion, the FDA test machines couldn't register it's components. 600 doctors showed up at the trial to testify on Dr. Koch's behalf, and in the process, represented thousands of patients that they said were cured by his methods. There were reports of Doctors being beaten up. Many newspaper articles were published on the subject, and congressmen read cures of humans and livestock into the congressional record.

After nine months of trial, he was acquitted. Tired of persecution, he moved to Rio de Janiero in 1953 to continue his work with that government's support. Back in 1935, the early formulations were being used in England, Belgium, and Brazil. By 1950 it was legally used worldwide, except in the U.S.. He died from poisoning, in Brazil, in 1967.

CATALYST MANUFACTURE AND PATIENT PREPARATION

Koch further explained: his Glyoxylide catalyst had to be made under ultra clean and pure conditions, and the ingredients had to be special, natural types. A patient was prepared by having him follow a special diet. Colonics were administered, as a necessary therapy, to clean out and restore the filtering mechanisms of the bowel. This was so that the released waste products, or oxidized toxins, would not be re-absorbed. Re-absorption of waste products could occur, due to a patient's inability to excrete them, because his colon was mucus-encrusted, or, plugged-up. The catalysts would cause the body to try and eliminate toxins, but if they couldn't get out through the colon, they would go back into circulation.

The oxidation starter was injected (2cc.) into the patient. Following injection, the patient at times shook violently for 3 or 4 minutes. If the patient was very toxic, he would experience some pain as the toxins were being oxidized and purged. If the patient was not too toxic, very little, or no discomfort followed. Koch's patients had no experience of any adverse effects. It was apparently completely harmless. In fact, any previous scar tissue (skin formed without enough oxygen) usually disappeared after the healing.

149

He produced many variations of his formulas, and kept improving them throughout his life. Many sources have sprung up claiming to be selling his compounds, but, unfortunately, some are just chemical mixtures, or weak versions. Koch stressed that his compounds are constantly changing, almost "alive", and are hard to duplicate. For example, some ingredients must come from mountain tops, and no plastic containers may be used during preparation.

As I stated, patient preparation, meaning a clean bowel, and diet were rigidly controlled. Otherwise the reaction would be used up quickly. "Crenation" tests, developed by Koch, were essential to monitor the oxygenating effectiveness of any therapy being used. It tells you where you are, and without using them, a doctor is not really using the Koch therapy.

CRENATION TESTS

I have paraphrased Koch's crenation test: a one percent solution of sodium chloride is mixed half and half with blood drawn from a fresh cut, on CLEAN, DRY skin, and a drop of this mixture is put on a slide. One then measures the amount of cells that crenate (shrivel up) within the first minute, and the number that do not, and those that not only stay round, but swell up instead. Speed is essential as in time they may all crenate. By being slow, one may get a false count.

The Crenation Theory: red blood cells have semi-permeable membranes. Each cell is filled by a certain amount of water that is held there, due to this osmotic membrane (permeable outer structure of the cell). If the salt solution can quickly draw cell water out through the membrane, the cell shrivels. Normally it should shrivel, as the outside 1% solution is hypertonic (has a different osmotic pressure) compared to the .85% normal osmotic pressure of the inside of the cell, so the inside solution moves to the outside. Therefore, when the cell refuses to shrivel, or worse yet, when it swells up, the osmotic pressure inside is too high. This means that the large protein molecules that should make up the cell are split into many smaller molecules. It also means that food molecules are present, that are not built up into the normal structures. In such situations, we have a picture of gross error.

Note: In the book, "Gary Null's Complete Guide To Healing Your Body Naturally", Mr. Null has a section on "Eating Right To Prevent Digestive Disorders" in which he states: "The way you masticate (chew)... is critical. Improper chewing also leaves food in chunks that are too large... when food is not broken down into small enough bits, it can enter the bloodstream as oversize particles. These particles cannot be used at the cellular level... during their prolonged stay in the blood, they are likely to elicit an immune response, through the activation of antibodies that do not recognize them as being compatible with the body's needs. Improper chewing thus can lead to... over-stimulation. of the allergic response." I suspect this was one of the warning signs Dr. Koch alluded to in his crenation test theory, when he found food particles in the blood cells that were not built up into the normal structures.

Here's a common error made by many trying to use the Koch formulas. Because they don't use the crenation tests, they give repeated shots, only days apart, trying to see what effects they're having. Koch almost never did this. He had the patient prepared and tested, and usually only gave one shot. Sometimes the patient was too toxic, and the first shot was blocked immediately, and in these rare instances, after more crenation testing, a second shot was given, but 14 days later. We sometimes think more is better, but in actuality, such a method is cycling the patient up and down, sending him on a "roller coaster" ride, when the body is probably over-stressed already from the disease. As Koch said in "The Survival Factor in Neoplastic and Viral Diseases": "One cannot give a bigger dose or repeat it beyond the ability of the patient to use it." and, "If the curative chemistry is started, it must be allowed to go as far as it can before the dose is repeated."

In the rare instances that the formula didn't work, Koch stated that it was because of a plugged up colon, unable to eliminate whatever toxins the "oxidation starters" gave the body to excrete. He also stated, that chelation therapies stop the Koch oxidation reactions from working, and the wrong diet also hinders it. Many, who don't have a serious illness, hear of the Koch formulations, and want to "try it". According to Dr. George Freibott (below), this would be a waste of the formula. Dr. Freibott cautioned, that one should not sensitize himself to it, but wait until it's needed. He also stated, that unless someone removes all the external causes of the illness, they would diminish the effectiveness of the treatment.

KOCH DIETARY RULES

I have paraphrased some of Koch's dietary rules during treatment. In his "Survival..." book, Koch said to avoid the following as being anti-oxygenating: radiation, oxides of nitrogen, antibiotics, frying pans and roasting ovens, fried or roasted foods where fats are used, aspirin and it's analogues, all coal tar products, insecticides, colorings and other food beautifying agents, selenium (a soil element found in grains grown in the middle west - corn, peas, lentils and wheat), sulfides, aluminum cookware and utensils, uncleaned fruits and vegetables, too much food, tea, coffee, mate, orange or lemon skins, salting, ice cream, soft drinks, poorly brewed beers, roasted peanuts (raw OK), combining proteins with carbohydrates during a meal, & lard.

Koch advocated that patients on his therapy eat these, as good oxygenators: fresh, clean, raw fruits and vegetables grown on selenium free soil, room temperature food instead of heated, snacking all day instead of eating 3 big meals, being a vegetarian, olive oil instead of butter, whole rye bread lettuce-tomato or bean or other vegetable sandwich (rye bread doesn't draw selenium out of the soil), slice of melon, apple, peach, bannana, or other fruit, a raw vegetable, carrot, onion, or chunk of cabbage snack, raw vegetable salad.

Note: According to the International Institute for Oxygen Therapies, the Koch Therapy and the Homozone Therapy (mentioned next), are not to be used with germanium or selenium treatments. The oxides are stripped away, and leave only the toxic elementals.

Excellent sources of information on Dr. Koch are the International Institute for Oxygen Therapies and BSRF. (See last section of this book). Koch's books and other works also may be purchased from: Cancer Book House 2043-OT N. Berendo, Los Angeles, CA 90027

KOCH'S WORK PARALLELS HOMEOPATHIC MEDICINE

Homeopathic medicine is experiencing something of a revival or rediscovery these days. Legal in the U.S. since 1832, Homeopathy was established two years before the American Medical Association (AMA), and at one point had 100 hospitals, 1,000 pharmacies, and 14,000 physicians. Homeopathy consists of the collected experience that: extremely dilute solutions of certain substances can cause (in a healthy person) the exact same symptoms as those that a diseased patient is already suffering. By administering these dilute, symptom-causing ingredients to a diseased patient, the Homeopathic physician causes the body to heal itself. Like affects like, in a rebound action. Usually applied in sugar pills, Homeopathic Medicine has now advanced to the point of computerized diagnostic machines that can scan a patient, and read out the exact needed dosages. Homeopathic medicine is mentioned here because the very diluted Koch catalyst formulas (some were 1 in 6 million concentration) amounted to homeopathic dilutions. This is the reason why many homeopathic remedies were analyzed as only "distilled water" by the FDA in the past.

Hector Delafuente assisted Dr. Koch when he was alive, and is quite knowledgeable about him and his work. he may be reached at P.O. Box 711-OT, San Carlos, CA 94070. Also, write BSRF (listed later) or the International Institute for Oxygen Therapies, below.

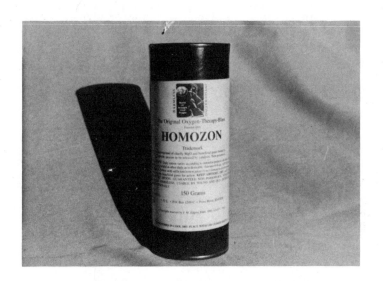

MODERN BLASS HOMOZONE FORMULATION

DR. F.M. EUGENE BLASS "OXYGEN-THERAPY-BLASS"

A contemporary of Dr. Koch, Dr. Blass published many works around 1929, and sold magnesium, calcium, and sodium based products that were reported to release ozone and hydrogen peroxide in the body. He also had preparations that one would bathe in, that allowed ozone/peroxide/nascent oxygen to be absorbed into the skin. His lab assistant saw him murdered (he was 88, and fit as a fiddle) in front of his house, by two men with clubs, around the same time as Dr. Koch.

In Dr. Blass's 1929 literature, we find the following quotes:

1. OXIDATION IS THE SOURCE OF LIFE AND HEALTH
2. IMPAIRED OXIDATION MEANS DISEASE
3. CESSATION OF OXIDATION IS DEATH

"DISEASE is: Impaired health due to impure vital fluids, a clogged up, and in its normal functions, hampered organism, giving food and lodging quarters for the various parasites, growths, etc., an unhealthy body!"

"LACK OF OXYGEN and minerals in the vital fluids (lack of health maintaining oxidation) is the true cause of disease, and lately has been admitted by medical experts to be the cause of cancer. This we have stated since 1922 and we also maintained since then, that through oxidation and mineralization of the diseased body this dreaded disease and all others can be avoided and eliminated if the laws of nature are honored and not misused."

"As long as the digestive tract is not cleaned, there is little or no chance for the active oxygen to reach, passing through the capillaries and blood vessels, the other, especially the extreme, parts or organs of the body...."

"Frequent stools (from use of the products) will cease as soon as the digestive tract is free of waste matters, then nascent oxygen (even of large and frequent doses of the preparations) will be available for the purification of the blood and lymph vessels and organs; a heavier urination will take place and is necessary to carry off the waste products of the oxidation process. As long as only Magazone or Homozone is used, watery stools will be present till the digestive tract is freed of waste matters. These stools are the logical result of oxidation (oxidation means changing solid waste matters into water and gas), it has nothing to do with diarrhea and does not weaken the body." (The Homozone just oxidizes waste so well, that it liquefies.)

Dr. Blass's products, (all TM) are all ozone or peroxide or nascent oxygen liberators: Magazone, a magnesium based powder product that oxygenates and loosens stools to promote intestinal cleansing. Calozone is calcium based, and is to be used when loose stools appear, and is an antilaxative. Macalzone is a mixture of Magazone and Calozone. Homozone is a stronger form of Magazone. San-O-Zone (and Pine San-O-Zone) is a sodium based powder that liberates ozone in external applications, as used in a bath. Oil "Mack", is a product extracted from Bavarian Alp Pines, grown on lime rocks at above 5000 feet altitudes.

The Koch Formulations worked by inducing the body to oxygenate itself with renewing amounts of antitoxin oxygen. The Homozone formulation has a different mechanism. Homozone releases, per can, many actual liters of oxygen, along with ozone, into the body via the stomach. Quite a package. It is a light, chalky tasting, white liquid, when mixed with water, and does release a large amount of oxygen immediately. This may be one of the most efficient oxygenators yet. The first teaspoon I tried had so much oxygen in it, that it made me giggle, and my head swoon.

More general, or detailed, scientific information on Dr. Blass, or Dr. Koch, etc., is available from: Dr. George Freibott, International Institute for Oxygen Therapies, P.O.B. 1360-OT, Priest River, ID 83856. Write Dr. Freibott for details. They are nonprofit (501K) medical missionaries, pledged to feeding the hungry, clothing the needy, and healing the sick. They have advocated Koch and Blass therapies for years, and just lost a building, equipment, and records, to a suspicious fire. They have just installed a computer BBS, so, if you have a computer and modem, you can dial in, and download oxygenation information.

A CLEAN BOWEL

Both Dr. Koch, Dr. Blass, and many others have maintained that healing is a process of proper oxygen and mineral intake, while removing the toxins. They have all stated, that to get enough oxygen and organic minerals into the body, the patient's bowel must be free from obstructions, as well as any old impacted fecal matter. These obstructions are commonly known to be hardened mucus-toxins that are clinging to, and impairing, the mineral and toxin exchange/transport function of the intestine walls. Again we have a controversy, as there is some current opinion around, that the colon is "only the equivalent of a hollow tube". Such a limited viewpoint is the opposite of a chart I once saw in a chiropractor's office. Apparently derived from thousands of years of oriental wisdom, The chart showed an "acupuncture" type point for every section of the colon, relating trouble in any of these sections to specific organs and areas of the body.

Consider this. The whole idea of eating, is to break the minerals down from the solid state they're in, in the food we eat, back to the "atom grouping" or ionic state. Mineral ions are what your body uses to build healthy cells. These ions are just like the mineral ions that come from the earth and go into the ionic exchange of a plant. These ions are taken up by the roots, and go into the "blood" of the plant, and the plant fluid distributes those minerals to the tissues to build cells. Our body works the same way. We've got to have minerals with the correct electrical charge, and those minerals have to come from an organic source, from the food we eat, to get back to the ionic state. That cycle is completed in the colon. If improperly digested food matter or unnatural chemicals stay in the colon too long, the body tries to protect itself from these substances with insulating secretions (mucus), and you've got a bunch of mucus caked up on the colon. If it stays there longer, you've created a favorable condition for anaerobic putrefying bacteria. Then your stools stink. You know your food is simply rotting inside you, instead of being absorbed back into your blood. You're stopping absorption and increasing putrefication, like in a stagnant swamp. Your bodily fluids, the lymph and the blood, are always dirty, as if your body was a car that never had it's air, fuel, or oil filters changed. A dirty machine doesn't function well, or for long.

To help you picture this better, let's follow some food, on it's approximately 30 foot journey through your body: first, you're supposed to take the time to chew your food into a liquid, combining it with enzymes from the mouth. Then it goes down to the stomach, where numerous acids and gastric secretions go through it, and then it goes into the small intestine. Here, more body fluids come through it, breaking the minerals down, from the solid state that they're in, back into the ionic state. Then, when it goes into your colon, it goes in as a liquid. The food in the first part of the colon is a liquid. A little higher up, it turns a semi-liquid. Up in the transverse part, it's a little more solid, a "semi-mush". From here it turns to "mush". It becomes semi solid in the descending colon, and then solid. Along the way, bodily fluids are leaving it, carrying the mineral ions back into your blood. Your body needs these minerals to build the strong genetic material of your cells.

Picture this: your body is trying to absorb these minerals back through the tiny sacs and projections covering the colon wall (as long as they're not all plugged up). That's where you're recycling your body fluids, your water in your body, that's where it's being filtered out. With that water that's being filtered, that's where you carry your minerals. Those minerals go through the colon walls, into to the lymphatic vessels and blood vessels that are just on the other side of the wall. The blood and lymph carry them to the cells. The minerals should be completing their cycle, and going back through the colon wall. If you fill your colon full of too much water, it washes these minerals out. You waste a big part of them. We have to let the colon do what it's supposed to do, recycling the body fluids, and absorbing the minerals. There's where you build your strong immune system, having and using enough minerals and oxygen to burn the cellular glucose, renew the cells, and remove the waste products of burning and renewing.

I found out, during an interview for this book, that Ed Goodloe, the president of Aerobic Life products, offers a product that reportedly solves the question of how to clean your bowel. Mr. Goodloe: "We've got a 10 day colon cleanse that allows you to eat normally when you do it, and you don't need a colonic machine or colonic board. You drink 5 ounces of aloe vera, from our own plantation in Brazil, with "special drink" in it, three times a day before meals. Between meals you drink 4 ounces of aloe vera with cranberry and papaya, 1 ounce of an herbal brew (aloe, camomile, golden seal, yellow dock, coconut oil, & potassium salt), and a tablespoon of powdered psyllium husks, (licorice, and hibiscus). Mix that up, drink it, and follow it with a glass of water. That does the trick."

"What happens, is that you actually stick new fecal matter to the old fecal matter when it gets in the colon, and the action of the colon literally strips it out. In around 3 days it'll probably come out, two feet or more long, all in one piece, when you first get on that cleanse - without a colonic. And then you aren't upsetting the normal absorption of minerals that go back through the colon wall into your blood. You'll see dark brown, spots, or tough, stringy stuff, 2 to 2 1/2 feet long, wrapped around, or attached to, the new fecal matter. That's the old fecal matter, all in one piece, sometimes coiled up like a snake. It gets the worms and parasites at the same time, because of some herbs we put in it." The 10 Day Colon Cleanse Kit is $76, and is available from: Aerobic Life Industries, Inc. 3045-OT So. 46th St., Phoenix, AZ 85040.

I've tried it. It did exactly what he said it would. It even instantly cleared up a chronic case of acne that a friend had. He assumes that the oxygenation products that he was using, were oxidizing his body's toxins, but his body was thwarted from sending the waste out through his colon. He saw the old waste come out. That, and no more acne, was proof enough for him that this worked.

156

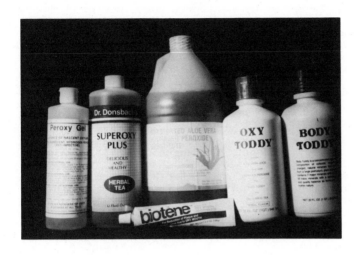

**PEROXY GEL, SUPEROXY PLUS, OXY TODDY,
BODY TODDY, BIOTENE, & OXYGENATED ALOE VERA**

HYDROGEN PEROXIDE PRODUCTS

When we speak of "hydrogen peroxide products," we assume the combination of something with hydrogen peroxide. A possible drawback to these combinations or mixtures, is that H_2O_2 and ozone are both such highly reactive substances, that when mixed with something, they will react with it. Still, I haven't heard of any cases where there were any problems with these blends, so this is still a theoretical consideration. The manufacturers claim there are no reactions because of the low concentrations used.

If there are indeed no reactions, I have a theory why. Most of the products - aloe, inner tree bark, natural sea minerals, etc. - that are being mixed with the H_2O_2, might be considered "live" or chemically close to it. This could be due to pH, cell enzyme titer, electron spin direction, electric characteristics, magnetic value, or some other process that needs to be found. Ingested, or absorbed, low concentrations of peroxide seem to only "target" diseased, dead, or dying cells, microbes and toxins, while leaving healthy cells untouched. Perhaps the substances being commercially mixed in with the peroxide aren't targeted (for oxidation) because they posses the characteristics we normally equate with life: "vitality" or "wholeness". No one has done enough lab work to prove this, so my making this statement isn't within the present day definitions of good science, it is strictly intuitive on my part.

157

Pure H_2O_2, by itself, dismutates (deactivates) spontaneously at a rate of about 1% per month. After several months, it may not be full strength. Dismutation is not slowed by refrigeration, but any chemical reactions are, so manufacturers advise you to refrigerate the blends, and use the freshest products. There have been reports that some of the products sitting on the shelf a long time have been tested, and found not at the advertised strength.

HYDROGEN PEROXIDE PILLS

There is a new method of Hydrogen Peroxide ingestion being used by Waves Forest and others. People are taking one pound of baking soda (or an inert culture powder) and mixing in 5 oz. of 35% H_2O_2. They let it dry, and put it in capsules. It is supposed to equal 4 drops of 35% per capsule, and they take 6 or 7 per day. They report that there is no nausea associated with this method of ingestion. I think that if it works, and doesn't react with the powder, or loose potency, it sounds great. The drawback with the peroxide liquids is their liquid form. If you spill them , they will oxidize or burn anything they touch, and they're bulky. Pills are dry and small. We will probably see this sold commercially.

ALOE VERA MIXED WITH HYDROGEN PEROXIDE

Because of some people's reluctance to drink dilute solutions of hydrogen peroxide, several entrepreneurs have developed mixtures to mask the bleachy taste. Usually, hydrogen peroxide is combined with Aloe Vera gels, and flavored to make a beverage. The unflavored ones are usually refrigerated (to thicken them), and rubbed into the hands or feet. These gels also have all the advantages of hydrogen peroxide absorption, with little risk of destroying friendly bacteria, since they bypass the stomach, and go directly into the body and bloodstream. **Users claim there is no nausea associated with this absorption method of ingestion.** I have found this to be true, but if I rubbed on an excessive amount, I would experience a slight "heartburn" feeling.

PEROXY GEL

A source of Nascent Oxygen, Peroxy Gel combines Aloe with red seaweed extract, natural glycerine, and 35% food grade hydrogen peroxide. Each teaspoon contains 20 drops of 35% H_2O_2. It is a gel when refrigerated, and a liquid at room temperature. Applied to the skin after bathing, it is directly absorbed, and bypasses the stomach. Skin absorption is less objectional than drinking it, and this method leaves the intestinal flora undisturbed. I have found that it delivered H_2O_2 just as well as drinking it. Exotic Herbal's sales literature states that Peroxy Gel may be taken internally for short term use, or brushed on the teeth. When I applied it, I could feel it sting very slightly, so I knew the potency was probably there. A 96-day supply, (1 16oz. bottle) is $15. They also have a product called "Peroxy Spray" that is a non-refrigerated alternative to their other products, and 35% Food Grade Hydrogen Peroxide, all 16 oz. at $15. Available from: Exotic Herbal Products, Inc., 29504-OT Evergreen Drive, Waterford, WI, 53185.

SUPEROXY PLUS ALOE VERA TONIC AND MIXTURES

Doctor Donsbach. Offers "Superoxy" in five "fabulous flavors", Cherry Berry (supposed to be the preferred one), Herbal Tea, Orange, Lemon Lime, & Plain. Each tablespoon contains 10 drops of 35% Food Grade Hydrogen Peroxide, - equal to 20 drops per ounce - made with a special blending process that inhibits aftertaste. They suggest ingesting 1/2 to one ounce, morning and night. This is the equivalent of 20 to 40 drops per day, of 35% peroxide. Dr. D's 32 oz., 1-quart size, is more liquid, and is slightly less potent, than Peroxy Gel, above. It is probably the easiest brand to find, in health food stores, since Dr. Donsbach already has his lines of distribution in place. Suggested retail $20.

OTHER DR. D'S PRODUCTS

Other Donsbach products are Pain Gel, a mixture of Hydrogen Peroxide and Dimethyl Sulfoxide (DMSO). Said to provide immediate pain relief, it comes in a 4 oz. size. Hydrogen Peroxide Tooth Gel, mint flavored, 4 oz., Sinus Nasal Spray, 3/4 oz. size, $3.95, and Ear Drops, 1/2 oz., $3.50. They also run The Hospital Santa Monica, in Mexico, that does Oxygenation Therapy, Ozone Therapy, and Hydrogen Peroxide infusions. They have a Video Cassette on the hospital for $10. DR. D'S Supplements, 323-OT E. San Ysidro Blvd. San Ysidro, CA.

OXY TODDY

Sold, since August of 1987, by multi-level marketing, OXY TODDY is a flavored product, a mixture of: aloe vera, 35% food grade hydrogen peroxide, Body Toddy (titrated, cold process, ancient sea bed minerals), and Pau D'Arco Tea. I have been assured, by the president of the Rockland Corporation, that experimental testing was done to find the least reactive and best tasting proportions of the various ingredients. Taken according to the directions on the label, each ounce has 20 drops of 35% H_2O_2 - the same as Donsbach's, and a pH of 4.5. Oxy Toddy was formulated by a chemist in California, in conjunction with Dr. Donsbach. It is said that Oxy Toddy has a good taste, because it has a different aloe than some others, plus they have their special tea flavoring. It comes in two flavors, Cranapple, and Herbal. $12.00 per quart at lowest dealer cost. (You must be signed up as a dealer first).

BODY TODDY

We've already discussed how important ionic minerals are to building strong genetic materials, cells, and immune systems. Here's an easily absorbable source. The original Body Toddy was discovered in 1931, and has been sold under the Body Toddy name for the past 6 years. It's a fantastic "organic" mineral concentrate, containing 6 vitamins, 22 amino acids, 7 major minerals, and 53 trace minerals. Altogether, 38,000 milligrams per quart, while some other brands are only 10,000 per quart. The pH is 2.8 to 3. Many diseases have responded to the reinstatement of a missing trace mineral. Minerals are the basic building blocks of our body, and are vital to oxygenation. Note: For an example, see the section on Germanium.

MINERALS USED FOR INJURIES

I have used these ancient sea bed minerals to kill infections I had, like a sore throat (gargle), or to immediately remove the pain and quickly heal any external skin cuts (one was right to the bone) by soaking in a solution of minerals and water. I have also wondered if a high oxygen level in the body might slow some wound healing. As I discussed in the first part of this book, hydrogen builds, and oxygen dissolves. Therefore the structure building process might be slowed by too much oxygen. Everything must be in balance. I seem to have experienced this, and the addition of these minerals to my diet sped up the wound healing process again. These minerals are still natural - compressed by nature - dried ancient plants that turned into sea beds, then the sea went away, leaving this deep mine shale in Utah just chock full of collodial minerals. These easily assimilated minerals, created by photosynthesis, are ten to twenty times smaller than minerals from rocks and soil.

Why this is not used clinically on burns, wounds, and infections I don't know, as it has always removed all pain and reduced my healing time by half. I am happy to find this product again, as my mineral source went out of business. Apparently these ancient sea bed natural mineral concentrates were produced under a number of private labels that came and went over the years.

Oxy Toddy and Body Toddy, plus water purification equipment, household cleaning products and others (even videos) are available in health food stores, or write: Elmer G. Heinrich, President, The Rockland Corporation, 12215-OT E. Skelly Drive, Tulsa, Oklahoma 74128.

BIOTENE HYDROGEN PEROXIDE GEL & TOOTHPASTE

Health food stores are starting to sell Biotene Toothpaste, which was formulated for anyone with "dry mouth". This toothpaste contains "the lactoperoxidase glucose oxidase antibacterial enzyme system". Glucose oxidase is an enzyme that has been used in Texas medical studies where it is injected directly into tumors, creates hydrogen peroxide out of body sugars, and gets rid of the tumor. In this toothpaste formula, the glucose oxidase and lactoperoxidase enzymes are carefully balanced to provide the production of hydrogen peroxide during brushing. The end result of the reaction produces hypothiocyante ions, which are able to penetrate the bacterial cell walls, to destroy these pathogens. Teeth get cavities from bacteria dissolving them, and can fall out because the gums become infected and recede, exposing the soft dentin (root) part of the tooth to bacteria and decay. When the dentin is decayed, the tooth will loose all support and fall out.

Sounds like a great formulation, and they back it up with clinical studies at the University of Rochester, and published medical studies of their system. The original formula had no fluoride in it, but it wouldn't sell. It seems that all the dentists will only recommend a product if it has fluoride in it, and won't let any product without fluoride to be exhibited at their trade shows and conventions. In order to survive, and sell product, Biotene had to add a small amount of sodium monofluoro phosphate, but I'm not worried about it. Another difference in their product, is their sweetener. Almost all toothpaste has saccharin in it for taste. It's on the labels, and the drawback is, that bacteria can grow in it. Biotene, however, solved that drawback by using Xylitol, a fruit juice sweetener found in strawberries, plums, and birch trees. It's natural, and bacteria don't like it. It tastes great, and leaves my mouth feeling "refreshed". Here's a good example of how to produce positive change, and not lose business.

Laclede, the corporation which sells Biotene, has developed their products, primarily, for people who have gone through radiation and chemotherapy. For example, elderly people, and people on medications, like antidepressants, that make their mouth very dry. Some, in the cases where radiation treatments have destroyed the salivary glands, have mouths so dry that they may wake up with their tongue stuck to the roof of their mouths. Biotene was first marketed to a specialty market, but their toothpaste may be used by anyone who wants to reduce bacteria in the mouth. They also "private brand" a clear hydrogen peroxide gel, under the Walgreens label, in the Walgreens national drugstore chain. The Academy of Dentistry For The Handicapped has endorsed their toothpaste, because it is harmless to swallow, as in the case of someone with Down's syndrome using it.

Biotene Toothpaste $4.95, Biotene Dental Chewing Gum $1.40, Walgreens Hydrogen Peroxide gel, and Oralbalance (artificial saliva) Gel $6 is produced by Laclede Professional Products, Inc. 15011-OT Staff Court, Gardena, CA 90248.

OXYGENATED ALOE VERA

The people at The Associates of International Health (AIH) have listened to hydrogen peroxide's negative press, being put out by certain competitive factions of hydrogen peroxide, and joined the fray, repeating some of it. AIH has decided to offer a hydrogen peroxide substitute. It's an aloe vera liquid, with oxygen forced into solution with it. Their position is this: "Hydrogen peroxide is OK., if someone has a serious illness, but we don't know enough about it yet, so everyone should take our product instead." As I have pointed out repeatedly, there is a window of demonstrated effectiveness with hydrogen peroxide that needs to be adhered to. I don't know of anyone who's been harmed by it, yet, and many have used it with benefit for years. Politics aside, this looks like a good idea. I don't know the shelf life or potency of their product, but the theory of the formulation is similar to the Pendell Water Oxygenator. Associates of International Health 12228 Venice Blvd. Suite 226-OT, Mar Vista, CA 90066.

PENDELL WATER OXYGENATOR

Mike Brown has come up with an invention that super saturates water with oxygen. The principle is the same found in nature, where you feel invigorated from swimming in white water, like the kind found under a waterfall. One of the reasons fish can't live long in tap water, is because it's so oxygen deficient. Nature has solved the problem of oxygenating water by tumbling it over rocks. Since water will only absorb oxygen if the water is one or two angstroms thick, meaning microscopically thin, Mike is selling a unit to optimize this action. It uses industrial tank oxygen (purchased from welding supply houses), and combines it with water sprayed over a packing material with a large surface area. Developed by mechanical engineer Larry Pendell, it causes so much oxygen to be absorbed, that a meter used to test water oxygen content was pegged off the scale. Drinking this water too fast can make your head swoon, it's so charged with oxygen. Mike Brown, PO Box 122-OT, San Marcos, CA, 92069

FLUORIDE?

Since we just mentioned some of the new hydrogen peroxide toothpaste brands, and then, Mike Brown's water treatment, and because we all brush our teeth and drink water, let's mention fluoride. Fluoride is a poisonous, industrial waste by-product from aluminum manufacture that needed a home, once upon a time. It ties directly into our "low oxygen levels lead to disease" theme, since a majority of our population ingests fluoride daily. Fluoride has been shown to reduce the body's ability to oxygenate. Oxygen intake into the system is an enzyme reaction, and fluoride has been proven to stop enzymes dead in their tracks. If you were to buy a can of it industrially, the can would come labeled with the "skull & crossbones" on it. Any toxin, even the poisonous mercury fillings in your teeth, can affect your oxygen uptake.

If you doubt what I'm saying, and reply: "Well, everyone uses fluoride, and they don't have any problems, do they?" then you simply haven't noticed the level of chronic degenerative disease around you. Let me quote for you, Pennsylvania Supreme Court Justice John P. Flaherty. He wrote this after holding a "very lengthy" series of judicial hearings on the fluoride issue:

"The evidence is quite convincing that the addition of sodium fluoride to the public water supply .... is extremely deleterious to the human body. A review of the evidence will disclose that there was no convincing evidence to the contrary... Prior to my hearing this case, I gave the matter of fluoridation little, if any thought, but I received quite an education, and noted that the proponents of fluoridation do nothing more than try to impugn the objectivity of those who oppose fluoridation. I seriously believe that few responsible people have objectively reviewed the evidence. If you are interested, I suggest that you review the 2,800 pages of testimony, and all the exhibits presented in this case." He issued an injunction against the use of fluoride.

The San Francisco Examiner newspaper did an article (10/6/83) on fluoride, and asks the pointed question: "If (fluoridation) is entirely safe, why has fluoridation been banned or abandoned in such enlightened European countries as Norway, Sweden, Austria, Belgium, Holland, Denmark, France, Italy, and West Germany?"

In the same article, the S.F. Examiner tells of Dutch MD, Dr. H. C. Moolenburgh and his colleagues, who studied it, and concluded that, "Fluoridation caused a low grade poisoning which stays beneath the surface in most people, but in some, and especially in those who's health is deteriorating, produces clinical symptoms."

Here are some medical references on mercury:

Subject: "**Immunosupression Produced by Lead Cadmium and Mercury**". Am. J. Vet. Res., 34 (11):1457-1458, 1973. "The significant aspect of the present study, is that chronic exposure to lead, cadmium, or mercury produces immunosuppression.."

Subject: "**Immune Dysregulation and Auto-Immunity Induced by Toxic Agents**". Druet, Hirsch, et. al. "As a consequence of immune dysregulation, auto-antibodies are produced, some of which are pathogenic significance. These results indicate that toxic agents (mercury) can induce abnormal lymphocyte interactions leading to auto-immunity as predicted by Allison."

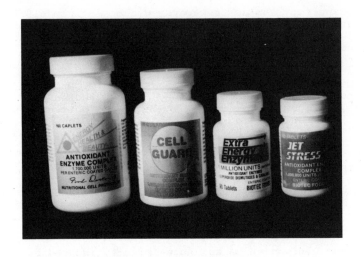

**CELL GUARD, ENERGY HEALTH & BEAUTY
WHEAT SPROUT ANTIOXIDANT ENZYME COMPLEXES**

SUPEROXIDE DISMUTASE
- IT CREATES HYDROGEN PEROXIDE

PROTEIN AND ENZYME IN ALL CELLS

Also known to veterinarians as Palosein (r), and to physicians as Orgotein (r), Superoxide Dismutase (SOD) is a protein, an enzyme, and known as erythrocuprein (since 1939). SOD, like Coenzyme Q-10, is in all body cells, and **fights the harmful free radicals in the body.** SOD **takes these radicals, and by dismutation (deactivation),** along with nature's catalase, **another dismuting enzyme, turns them first, into stable oxygen and hydrogen peroxide, then into water and oxygen.** When we speak of SOD, we are referring also to calalase, as either one without the other is toxic. SOD is the fifth most abundant body enzyme.

LOW LEVELS OF SOD MAY CAUSE PROBLEMS

When harmful free radicals are left unchecked, they attach to supporting tissue collagen. This process makes our tissues stiff, our skin wrinkled, and causes deposits to form on the arterial walls. The process is very similar to my description of the solidifying effects of hydrogen. Many say that because SOD removes free radicals, it removes a major cause of aging.

The use of SOD is becoming widespread. Even Harper's Bazaar magazine ran an article calling SOD, "The Live Longer Pill". Seattle Slew, the racehorse, went on to win The Kentucky Derby, and the Triple Crown, after being injected with SOD.

164

ARTHRITIS

If SOD is continued, the arthritis symptoms will disappear.
                    - Dr. W. Huber, of Diagnostic Data, Inc.

"It appears that natural SOD will relieve the morning stiffness, pain, and swollen joints in about 85% of arthritis patients. SOD should be of benefit, if sufficient amounts are taken, to replace cellular production deficiencies due to age or stress. A million units a day would be an absolute minimum for anyone over 30 years.."

"...a remarkable substance for treating arthritis, which affects more than 22 million Americans.... It will relieve the sufferings of millions of people!" - Dr. James L. Goddard, The former Assistant Surgeon General of the United States.

AGING

"If we could supplement the two million units per day of superoxide dismutase and catalase, that is no longer produced in the cells of a sixty year old, we would see a remarkable change for the better in the health of millions of older Americans." - Dr. A.W. Huber.

"The therapeutic possibilities are mind boggling, for we may have in our grasp, a system of enzymes which allow us to slow down aging, and to prevent, and reverse, a long list of degenerative diseases." - Dr. Milton Fried, Atlanta

HEART

St. Louis University Researchers said that the use of SOD after heart attack appears to assist in the restoration of damaged heart tissue.

RADIATION

Others have tried it, to reverse the harm from radiation treatments, including sunburn, VDT, microwaves, and fallout. Dr. Donsbach has suggested, if you've been exposed to nuclear radiation, "then you might want to eat it like popcorn! (it can't hurt you)." He used it on his own daughter, after she had radiation treatments for Oat Cell Cancer. Now she has no cancer or radiation effects. Radiation creates free radicals and SOD deactivates them.

"It is ironic that radiation can convert oxygen, essential for life, into toxic substances which can destroy us."

"...a sturdy little organism, a bacterium called Radiodurans, that thrives inside operating nuclear reactors. Guess what's inside these bacteria? The highest levels of SOD/CAT (and other antioxidant enzymes) ever measured!"

"In recent tests by the Swedish government on people with radiation sickness from the Chernobyl accident, these enzymes were the only ones which produced noticeable relief."

- Lita Lee, Ph. D.

NATURALLY OCCURRING SOD

These supplements have proven very helpful for arthritis and other geriatric degenerative problems in my practice as well as in the practice of other veterinarians throughout the country. SOD - catalase supplements are harmless. - Dr. M. Lemmon, D.V.M. Holistic Animal News, PO Box OT1, Seattle, WA, 98109

Water-soluble SOD is extremely similar, whether in man, or plant, and is said to be universal in all plants that grow in oxygen, and the greener the plant, the more SOD. Found everywhere in nature, SOD is predominant in the greenest plants: kale, spinach, collards, comfrey & broccoli. It is also on the shelves of health food stores, and can be ordered from. Dr. D'S Supplements, 323-OT E. San Ysidro Blvd, San Ysidro, CA. 619/428-8585. Credit goes to him for some of the above ideas in his book, "Superoxide Dismutase."

NEW SUPER SOD

It is also available in health food stores from various manufacturers. One example is Solgar. They have a formula of SOD that also has catalase in it, necessary to break down the H_2O_2 created by SOD. Catalase is the chief enzyme that breaks down hydrogen peroxide. Even more exciting, however, is the new generation of "high unit dosage" SOD developed by botanists, from Indian wheat sprouts. **Each tablet is equal to a square foot of wheat sprouts, 2 inches high, or 8 bottles of regular SOD found in the stores.** The regular kind had only, approx., 2,000 units in each pill.

HIGH POTENCY SUPER OXIDE DISMUTASE COMBINED WITH H_2O_2

Hydrogen Peroxide works by releasing, "good" free radical singlet oxygen into the body. Ozone also creates radicals. This, so far, hasn't been a problem if the immune system works well. If not, then some have recommended the use of the food product complex, super oxide dismutase tablets. This is to be sure that any extra free radicals left over from the hydrogen peroxide reactions - in other words, any peroxide created radicals that didn't combine with any "out of balance" elements - are balanced out, themselves, before they cause any harm.

Some have observed that ozone therapy works better without these antioxidant enzymes being taken during the treatments, but used afterwards, to protect from any free radical chain reactions. The observations suggest anyone using H_2O_2 or ozone might want to rotate their use with these enzymes.

AGE DECREASES NATURAL SOD PRODUCTION

When we get older our bodies produce approximately 3.4 million units of SOD daily, while a child creates approximately 5.1 million units. One tablet of the new antioxidant food enzyme complex with SOD yields, with biological activity, the equivalent of 1.5 to 1.7 million units. Taking a few tablets of this substance will theoretically give an older person approximately the same amount of daily available antioxidants as they produced as a child.

ANTIOXIDANT SUPER SOD FOOD COMPLEXES

Super SOD complexes contain approximately 28% SOD, 28% glutathione peroxidase, 28% methionine reductase, and 16% catalase. A Dr. Rothschild, MD, Ph.D., MS, has done some testing, found that there is a high level of "biological activity" with these complexes made from sprouts. Biological activity is an FDA term, referring to the action of a substance within a living organism, rather than as static test tube reactions. The biological activity level is so high, that during a double blind study, up to 30 days after no longer taking the product, certain antioxidant enzyme levels were still increased from 90 to 100% over the day when they first started!

Contrast this with normal food digesting enzymes. Their activity stops in a few hours. Same with injectable food-complexed SOD, it mostly disappears right away. When in a whole food matrix, as in the new Biotec food complexes, it is able to incorporate itself into living tissue and be preserved, instead of being oxidized. This is also due to another process called "enzymogen activation". These enzymogens are the precursors or starters of bodily enzyme production. The complex, being incorporated into living tissue, is stored as the substances needed to make the enzymes, when called upon by the body, as it detects harmful free radicals. The unit dosages, stated on the labels of these products, reflect the biological activity, not the chemical activity.

This new form of SOD/enzyme complex is produced by taking special wheat sprouts, and stressing them during their growth phase. To protect themselves, the sprouts produce all the antioxidant enzymes necessary to fight the formation of increased free radical levels. When eaten, these antioxidant free radical fighters are easily incorporated into our body tissues because they are natural. In other words, through a special process of plant genetics, the wheat sprouts have a high level of enzyme activity and content, and are in their own wholefood matrix, providing all the nutritional cofactors necessary for efficient biological effect.

Consider these examples: people who work in nuclear power plants have been tested, and show higher levels of SOD in their bodies. Bacteria growing within nuclear reactors have an extremely high level of SOD. Both instances show how nature will attempt to protect an organism against harmful free radical formations.

BIOTEC

The only company presently selling this form of food complex is Biotec. Biotec sells an antioxidant enzyme complex product made from special Indian wheat, claimed to be 700 times more potent than the average SOD found in stores. If taken while using H_2O_2, but far enough apart, so they don't cancel each other, it has been theorized that the two work together as a "dynamic duo", cleaning out the body, preventing free radical damage (such as premature aging), boosting the immune system, and removing disease. Did that get your attention?

The aim is to get the oxygen into the system in a form the body can utilize, and at the same time protect the basic healthy tissue of the system from the oxidative process, by using enzymes. There have been ancedotal reports attesting that this is how this combination works, and more research is needed to explore these fantastic combinations.

Supposedly, the only reported negative might be the rare instance of someone having some sort of wheat allergy that could flare up, since the taking of this SOD complex is eating dried compressed special wheat sprouts. Usually, someone with a wheat allergy already knows it.

The manufacturer of this high potency complex, Biotec Foods, sells it: to multi level marketers as "Food Doctor's Energy Health And Beauty Antioxidant Enzyme Complex", to health food stores as "Biotec's Cell Guard", "Runners Edge", and "Anti-Stress Enzymes", to veterinarians under "Biovet International", and to health professionals as "Biomed Food's AOX-PLX". The company is located in Hawaii. The U.S. distributor, Zane Baranowski, is at 597-OT Glenwood Cutoff, Scotts Valley, CA 95006. Available by mail order through: U.S.S. Goodship, P.O. Box 1116-OT, McMinnville Oregon. 97128. Health-Tec, 208K-OT E. Alma, Mt. Shasta, CA 96067. The prices may seem high, around $35, but as we said, one tablet is equal to about eight bottles of the old SOD, so cost that out in comparison.

"Evidence of the effectiveness of enzymes taken orally is beginning to overwhelm skeptics. Much of the evidence comes from many years of studies performed in West Germany, Switzerland, Austria, Italy and Mexico. Many of these studies show proteolytic enzymes, when taken orally, demonstrating benefits against circulating immune complexes, rheumatic disorders, and auto-immune diseases. More recently, studies conducted with antioxidant enzymes are beginning to objectively confirm clinical successes in veterinary and medical practices."

- Peter R. Rothschild, MD, Ph.D. Biochemistry, MS Quantum Physics. Author of 16 scientific books, 36 articles, and nominated for the Nobel Prize, in Physics, in 1986.

CO ENZYME Q10

CAN WE ADD 50% TO A LIFETIME AND LOOSE WEIGHT TOO?

There has been a surge of interest in CoQ10, and even such magazines as <u>Muscle and Fitness</u> are doing articles on it. Here's the story on it:

Every cell in our body has the co-enzyme Q10 in it. Also known as Ubiquinone. Ubiquinone, comes from the word ubiquitous, or, "existing everywhere at the same time", and quinone - a coenzyme. "Q10", means it has 10 isoprene units in a long molecular chain of 50 atoms arranged in ten groups of five atoms each. Q10 is believed to be the only CoQ of prime importance to man. A crystalline substance discovered in the 50's, it has the ability to "transfer" electrons as needed, from molecule to molecule. The human body will not function without it, and can only get it from food.

Enzymes are protein substances found in every living thing, and are made up of a protein part, and a vitamin or mineral part (the cofactor). The vitamin part is called the coenzyme. Being right there next to the "action", it supplies quick energy to the cells.

NECESSARY TO CELL "IGNITION"

Here's how. Within each tiny cell, are still smaller components called mitochondria. CoQ supplies the mitochondria the igniting "spark" and nutrients, that permit energy production. Without these "sparks" or igniting inputs, there is no respiration, no life. If these coenzymes are in a deficient condition, then only some of the cells are working, or oxygenating. That means the energy levels drop (or cease) in the rest, leaving them ripe for infection, mutation, or elimination.

Our food and air must be burned within the body to create energy. You can see how coenzymes tie into oxygenation and the creation of this energy. They function as biochemical catalysts. The word enzyme, comes from a Greek word meaning "an element or influence that works subtly to enliven the whole".

POSSIBLE WEIGHT LOSS

"Q10 may accelerate weight loss in some obese patients" Some scientists did a study proving it, quoted from <u>Search For Health</u>, Vol 1, #3, quoting a medical bulletin for physicians.

MANIPULATES OXYGEN IN CELLS

"CoQ has the ability to manipulate Oxygen. It can add or take away oxygen from a given biochemical combination, moving oxygen in or out of the mitochondria. It can increase oxygen levels when necessary, and reduce them if they threaten to reach toxic levels". And, "Although still speculation, the connection does seem obvious between the proven immune boosting benefits of

CoQ10 and the type of immune boosting being sought in AIDS research and therapy".
Emile G. Bliznakov, M.D., President and Scientific Director of the Lupus Research Institute, in "The Miracle Nutrient Coenzyme Q10"

FOUND IN MAJOR ORGANS AND LINKED WITH HEART DISEASE

The greatest amount of our internal CoQ10 is found in our heart and liver. Historically, it was first found in the heart by Dr. Karl Folkers. This is significant to us, as the heart doesn't get cancer. Some researchers now think that a decline of CoQ10 goes hand in hand with heart disease. Research has shown that cardiac patients have much lower CoQ10 levels than healthy people. - Folkers, Nadhanavikit and Mortensen, Proceedings of the National Academy of Sciences, 1985, 62, 901-904.

If you want to have some fun, ask a doctor why no one ever has heart cancer. I say fun, but it's sad they never even think of asking the question. CoQ10 is widely prescribed as a heart medicine in Japan, but not in the United States.

This information also ties into the work of Dr. Koch, who's famous "oxidation starter" was first patterned after heart area chemicals for that very reason. After Q10 was discovered, Dr. Koch spoke of it thusly. It's a real mind stretcher, so read it slowly.

KOCH SPEAKS OF CO-Q10

"Their structures are essentially carbonyl groups activated by conjugation with double bonds of ethylenic linkages...in the case of quinones the double bonds are not altered, and reversal with return of function is possible. Thus coenzyme Q can function as a co-enzyme over and over again as an electron transfer agent."

"The quinone structure is also admirably adapted to such function so as to meet the requirements of specificity in oxidation-reduction potential and for selecting the specific materials it will react with in each particular cell activity."

"The substituents placed about the quinone's double bonds give the steric advantages and hindrances required for specific reactions and for elevated or depressed negativity and oxidation-reduction potentials of the carbonyl groups."

"Today...the position of the free radical which can now be proven by electron spin resonance techniques is demonstrated as fundamental to all living processes." - The Survival Factor In Neoplastic and Viral Diseases. Koch.

REMOVES FREE RADICALS

CoQ10 can add or remove oxygen from other substances in the body, and recent research proved it to be a strong antioxidant. - Lenaz, Coenzyme Q, New York: John Wiley, 1985. My research efforts lead me to suspect, that it regulates oxygen transport, plus or minus, and is not strictly "anti" anything.

IN LIVERS

Our livers produce it from Q7 but loose the ability to produce it as we get older. The liver converts all other CoQ's to CoQ10, but the older you get, the less of this conversion your body can make. Therefore, everyone over 35 may be deficient. It is said that when your body levels drop 30% below the norm, you may be open to degenerative effects. It has also been suggested that a deficiency of CoQ10 accelerates aging, while an increase promotes youth. In one study by Bliznakov, Q10 supplemented old lab mice had their lives extended 50%!

IN FOODS

Foods high in natural CoQ10 are: mackerel, sardines, cereals (esp. brans), nuts, dark green vegetables (spinach and broccoli), soybeans and rapeseed, soy and sesame oils. The Japanese use fermentation processes to produce it for the mass market, where millions use it in doses of 10 to 30 mg. a day. Reportedly, it may take up to three months of Co-Q10 ingestion to saturate deficient tissues.

COMMERCIAL PREPARATIONS

You have to be inquisitive about the commercial preparations available. The original Japanese version comes in a little yellow pill form. Some capsules are filled with inexpensive quinones in order to give them the yellow color, but are not the quality or potency claimed. Calcium or magnesium fillers are said to "have the wrong electricity" by Dr. Hans Nieper of Germany. The best filler is a very small amount, and is chemically and electrically inert. Emulsifying it is an added unnecessary step.

It is available in health food stores and from APW 800/522-4279 (which supplies it with an audited assay), Nutricology 800/545-9960, Biogenesis 800/ 345-4152 & Exotic Herbal Products 414/534-4200. Please mention this book, as I am trying to measure it's reach.

GERMANIUM

Organic Germanium is a prevalent trace mineral element that acts as a semi-conductor, entering into our biochemical equations by balancing the oxygen content of the cells - an "oxygen carrier". It's proper name is Bis-betacarboxyethyl germanium sesquioxide, and as a mineral, it helps conduct the body bioelectricity. It is a clear to white crystalline, odorless powder.

The key activity of germanium appears to be the added oxygenation made available by the special sesquioxide chemistry, wherein three oxygen molecules are readily available for the oxidation mechanisms. Dr. Kazuhiko Asai, a Japanese chemist, perfected a process of producing crystalline germanium, after finding the highest concentrations of it in medicinal plants. He says he cured his own advanced arthritis with it, by taking 250 to 1500 mg/day, orally. He also states that, when the blood is too acidic, germanium is not effective. This points up the need for a whole systems approach to oxygenation. The Japanese have germanium baths (osmosis through the skin), and it's only in the U.S., that we mainly use it in injections and pills. It is FDA approved, as a trace mineral food supplement.

Germanium spares oxygen, and chelates toxic substances out of the body, especially mercury, cadmium, and lead. By regulating our cellular oxygen levels, it enhances the immune system, as has already been explained in this book, affecting a wide range of anaerobic disease.

It's small size permits rapid diffusion across membranes... It's active site is probably at specific sites on the respiratory chain in mitochondria, increasing the efficiency of electron transport to oxygen. - Tsutsui, M. J. Am. Chem. Soc. 8287-8289, 1976.

"Organic germanium restores the normal function of T-cells, Blymphocytes, natural killer cell activity, and the numbers of antibody-forming cells. Studies indicate that this compound has unique physiological activities without any significant side effects. Organic germanium has the ability to modulate alterations in the immune response." Journal of Interferon Research #4, 1984.

"Organic germanium-treated test animals show an inhibitory effect against certain tumors in such a way that would suggest that the effect is the result of increased macrophage (similar to white blood cells in immune system) activity. 'Gan To Kagaku Ryoho' #12, Nov. 1985 Japan.

"The antitumor action of organic germanium appears to be related to its interferon-inducing activity." Tohoku Journal of Experimental Medicine #146, May 1985.

What we have is another oxygenation booster, and immune system repairer. Look at this quote: "Organic germanium restores the impaired immunoresponses in aged mice." International Archives of Allergy #63, 1980.

"Patients receiving the compound have shown virtualy no metastasis. (Metastasis is the transitional spreading of cancer to other parts of the body.)... If the (spreading) can be prevented, cancer can be stopped with a massive attack on the primary lesion (injury)...After a dose of organic germanium, within a short time, the amount of oxygen in the body is not only greatly increased, but *dehydrogenation takes place, and poisonous matter is rendered nonpoisonous, and in about 20 hours is thrown out of the body. Since germanium does not remain in the body, there is absolutely no toxicity and no harmful side effects...*" Dr. Asai, "Miracle Cure; Organic Germanium."

When the blood is too acidic (too much carbolic or uric acid, for example) germanium has a much harder time oxygenating the body. The stabilized oxygenation products, like Aerox and Aerobic 07, (See following sections) allegedly can clean the blood enough to let germanium work. So, again, we see that health is a whole systems approach.

It has been reported by insiders that true germanium is expensive, and there have been imitations, even labeled "Asai germanium", when his institute didn't make it. So be inquisitive. Tests have shown that only the Germanium Sesquioxide produced in Japan under the supervision of the Japanese Food and Drug Administration is free of contamination from Germanium Dioxide, a far cheaper but toxic substance. I cannot personally attest to any product's origins or purity.

Natural germanium is found in many plants, especially garlic, ginseng, aloe vera & alfalfa. Most of these have been used as healing agents since civilization began. Is germanium why? It is also naturally occurring on the shelves of health food stores.

IIOT warns against using germanium or selenium if a patient is undergoing Koch or Homozone Therapies, as they strip the "oxides" away, leaving the toxic elemental.

Germanium sesquioxide can be ordered from: APW, P.O.Box 3048-OT, Iowa City, IA 52244. APW sells only the exact germanium used by Dr. Asai's clinic in Japan. Some concerns sell what they call "Asai germanium", but it's not his. APW also sells a copy of Dr. Asai's book "Miracle Cure; Organic Germanium" for $17. It is the definitive reference on the subject.

Germanium is also available from: The Warta Company, P.O.Box 407-OT, Delano, MN 55328. Allergy Research Group, 400-OT Preda St., San Leandro, CA 94557 (They also have medically documented product fact sheets). The Stephen A. Levine, Ph.D. formulas, are available from: Nutricology, 400-OT Preda St., San Leandro, CA 94577. Dr. Donsbach's Supplements, 323-OT E. San Ysidro Blvd, San Ysidro, CA. Credit goes to Dr. Donsbach for some of the above quotes in his $1 book "Germanium, Ge-132"

THIOCTIC ACID (THIOX)

Also known as lepoic acid, thioctic acid is a non-toxic nutrient cofactor included in this work because of it's ability to oxidize serious poisons, such as mercury toxemia, and "destroying angel" mushroom poisoning. It's a special liver detoxifier. The liver is the body's factory for production of enzymes hormones and proteins. If toxins build up in the liver, it can't do it's job. In one study, at the National Institute of Health (NIH), 4 out of 5 mushroom poisoning victims were cured.

Only a trace amount can be isolated in tissue. Essentially, it helps metabolize liver toxins. Physicians have demonstrated a strong antitoxic action against chronic poisoning by "mercury chloride, arsenobenzoles, carbon tetrachloride and analine dyes". Experiments adding thioctic acid to algae showed a quantum yield of oxygen production by over 50%.

APW states that a physicians report lists the following "clinical indications" for the use of thioctic acid: Chemical Hypersensitivity Syndrome, Heavy Metal Toxicity, Diabetic Neuropathy, Chronic Aggressive Hepatitis, elevated liver enzymes; other chronic liver diseases, Peripheral Neuropathy, withdrawal symptoms from glucocorticoids, Alcoholism and narcotic addiction, as well as various poisonings."

All of the above from the APW newsletter "Search For Health". APW sells THIOX, their own brand of thioctic acid. APW, P.O.Box 3048-OT, Iowa City, IA 52244.

TAHEEBO/PAU D'ARCO/LAPACHO TREE

This tree fixes crystals of high oxygen content within it's bark. The bark has been used for centuries by the locals to prevent and reverse illnesses. It is available in the US as an herbal tea in health food stores.

VITAMINS E & A "ANTIOXIDANTS?"

Vitamin E tremendously reduces the body's need for oxygen. Mattill, H.A., Nut. Rev., 10,225,1952 Telford, E.A., et al., Air U Sch. Aviation Med. Rep. 4 Project 21,1201 1954. Zierler, M., et al., Ann. NY Acad. Sci. 52, 180,1049. Houchim, O.B. et al., J. Biol. Chem. 146, 309,313,1942 De Nicola, P., Inter. Congress Vit. E 1955 Shute, E.V., Inter. Congress Vit. E 1955 Jessen, K. E., et al., Acta Path. Microbiol. Scand. 29, 72, 1951

Without enough vitamin E, Vitamin A is quickly used up by oxygen. - Moore, T. Biochem. J., 34, 1321,1940.

It protects essential fatty acids, carotene, Vitamin A, B vitamins (indirectly) and the pituitary, adrenal, and sex hormones from being destroyed by oxygen. Mattill, H.A., Nut. Rev. 10, 225, 1952 Moore, T. J. Nut. 65, 185, 1958 Pazcek, P.L., et al., J. Biol. Chem. 146, 351, 1942 Beckman, R., Inter. Cong. Vit. E, 202, 1955

"Pain caused by lack of oxygen, common in the heart, eyes, legs, feet, or any tissue where the circulation is decreased by fatty deposits, is often markedly relieved in a few days after Vitamin E is added to the diet." Shute, E.V., and Shute, W.E., Alpha Trocopherol in Cardiovascular disease, Ryerson Press, Toronto, Canada 1954. Tolgyes, S., et al., Canadian Med. Assn. Journal 76,730, 1957

RETIN-A

There's a lot of interest in Retin-A, one of the retinoids from vitamin A, that gets rid of old, wrinkled skin and grows new, soft, supple, non-wrinkled skin in it's place. It is said to repair DNA, and grow many new blood vessels. These new blood vessels supply life-giving oxygen to the cells, allowing them to grow in beauty.

"ANTIOXIDANT" A MISNOMER?

Vitamins A&E, are often labeled, by well meaning people, as "antioxidants". By this labeling, oxidation (oxygen), the process of energy creation and life, is thereby inferred to be causing harm, or premature aging, or something. We are told we must take "antioxidants" to stop the "toxic free radicals." Might I propose that this admonition is a current "science fashion" and it would be better to call them "oximodulators".

"Oxygen is the greatest giver and receiver of electrons in the elemental world, so oxygen is almost always involved in free radical chemistry." Search For Health Vol 1, #3.

The facts and documentation I have assembled for you here in "O_2xygen Therapies - A New Way Of Approaching Disease", plainly show that the label, "anti-" shows us only half the story. When oxygenation exceeds it's window of usefulness, we can slow down the reactions- bring them into balance. This is not the same as "anti" or preventing all action. The same applies to the recent "all free radicals are bad" approach. As I have shown, it's only some of them that are bad, and those might be actually quite natural and neutral, except that the other side of the equation - the "good" ones are missing, and can't balance them out.

These missing parts of the human biochemical equation, and how researchers are adding them, to rebalance the equation, are the subject of this book. In all my studies of healing and spiritual systems, the one point that constantly impresses me, is the way that Nature will always seek balance. It has also been said "nature abhors a vacuum." This is another way of stating it. When there is too much of something, or not enough, when either are compared to the whole, something "happens" to reestablish balance.

Perhaps we should consider this: when viewed from a detached, "whole systems" perspective, everything that happens to you, is somehow Nature seeking balance. It matters little, to The Universe, if you can understand this, because it just keeps operating under it's prime directives and immutable laws, until you do. Time is on It's side, and if you consider our life's strivings, it makes sense that we are seeking balance ultimately as individuals. Whole and minute systems are mirrored in each other. We only view them from different points on the ascending spiral of life, and proclaim them separate.

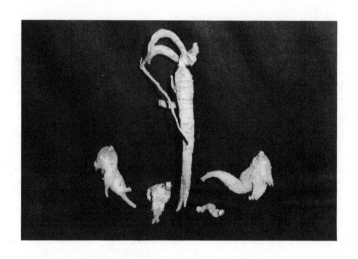

WILD NORTH AMERICAN GINSENG

GINSANA & GINSENG

Ginsana is a ginseng product, that a trusted friend of mine likes. I don't have any experience with it myself. I have, however, used Ginseng, and like it. Mankind has used ginseng for over 4,000 years, to build physical endurance, mental alertness, harmonious balance, and overall well-being. Ginseng falls into the category of a "bitter herb". Like all bitter herbs, it contains more chlorophyll and alkalines. These substances are what contain the oxygen, the more bitter they are, the more oxygen they contain. Ginsana (r) or G115 (r), unlike the ginseng root itself, has equal ginseng extract potency, from dose to dose. The retail price reflects the amount of special processing needed to achieve this uniformity of dosages.

There have been many clinical studies of ginseng. Two areas fit into our oxygenation theme: oxygen uptake and pulmonary function. Both these areas have importance to athletes and anyone who is ill. Oxygen uptake is a measure of how well we utilize oxygen during work, and the more we can utilize, the more endurance we have. Pulmonary function is a measure of how well we breathe.

As you have already probably surmised, the studies showed both processes were enhanced significantly by using Ginsana (r). Oxygen uptake increased in one study group from 3,900 (milliliters) to 4,500 in 12 weeks. Pulmonary function (FEV_1 - Forced Expiratory Volume and FVC - Vital Capacity) was similarly increased. FEV_1 went from 4,600 to 4,800. FVC went from 5,600 to 6,000.

All figures are close approximates. The placebo groups had virtually no change.

- E. Dorling et al.: Do ginsengosides influence the performance? Results of a double blind study. Notabene Medici, 10, 5: 241-246 (1980).

- I. Forgo/G. Schimert: The duration of effect of the standardized Ginseng extract G115 in healthy competitive athletes. Notabene Medici, 15, 9: 636-640 (1985).

Chewing the ginseng root, or drinking it's extract, has always given me a feeling of being more "alive", without the artificial up and down stimulation of caffeine, while apparently increasing my immunity and recuperative powers. As the above studies showed, oxygenation was increased with ginseng use. Ginsana use is a way to receive measured doses. Ginsana is available from Ginsana USA Corp. 50-OT Maple Place, Manhasset, NY 11030.

H_2O_2 LIQUID STERILIZATION

From Henley's 20th Century Book of Formulas, Processes & Trade Secrets, 1956 Books, Inc. NY:

Mix 1.3%, by volume, of H_2O_2 into milk, and shake well. Heat for 5 hours at 122 to 125 degrees F, in well closed vessels. Upon cooling, the milk will retain it's taste and freshness for 1 month.

Father Willhelm says to put 12 drops of 35% in a quart.

Preservation of drinks. 2 1/2 Fluidrachms of commercial Peroxide of Hydrogen per quart of syrups, wine, beer, cider, or vinegar.

Also, a test for bacteria in water. Put a few drops of H_2O_2 in water, and if it produces bubbles, then, the H_2O_2 is decomposing bacteria. Sometimes the gas production is quite brisk.

ELECTRON/OXYGEN TRANSPORT SUBSTANCES

STABILIZED ELECTROLYTES OF OXYGEN PRODUCTS

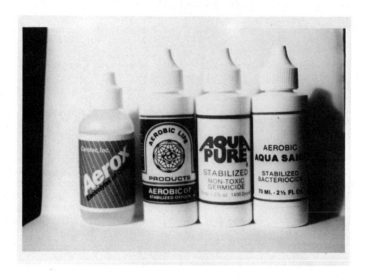

AEROX, AEROBIC 07

CHLORINE DIOXIDE

The following liquid commercial formulations are what's known as variations on the chlorine dioxide (peroxide) theme. They deliver oxygen to the body, but each in a different way than hydrogen peroxide, and from each other. Some of these formulations are based upon sodium peroxide, and some chlorine peroxide. People question whether they leave any chlorine residue, the Aerox people state their product doesn't. Chlorine dioxide gas is a tremendous oxidizing gas, it will kill any parasites or even humans, depending on the amount. The right amounts, in the right formulations, are great oxygenators. But, too much can kill. Again our "window of effectiveness" comes into view. These formulations have been the basis of some commercial products here in the U.S.. The ones I know of are discussed below.

They are alkaline, and similar in effect to Hydrogen Peroxide, but are more stable, and instead of releasing gas in the stomach, they react with stomach acids, and release "molecular" oxygen. Somehow, this averts any nauseous feelings, and they seem to "go deeper", and have almost no taste. Unlike hydrogen peroxide, they also do not require the action of the enzyme catalase, because stomach acid activates them. When they release molecular oxygen upon contact with the stomach acid, they also release just enough of a minute amount of chlorine gas, to kill stomach bacteria, but apparently not enough to hurt us.

178

There doesn't seem to be any strong "cleansing reactions" with their use. The only negative seems to be, the rare someone, who is missing the enzyme "glucose 6 phosphate dehydrogenase (G6PH)". If you're one of these people, you probably know it already. These products are more costly and complicated to produce than hydrogen peroxide, due to the manufacturers having to combine ingredients under specific temperatures, and pressures, repeatedly, until an end result is produced that is unrecognizable from the ingredients. The manufacturers say, that the advantages of these products are reflected in their cost.

AEROBIC 07

First, there is a product called "an aqueous solution of non-toxic stabilized chlorine dioxide", or Aerobic 07, private branded as EQO_2, and others. From the literature of Aerobic Life Products, the manufacturer: "Stabilized oxygen is a high concentrate of oxygen - oxygen in the molecular form... Stabilized Oxygen actually puts oxygen in the blood, without the process of breathing. It cannot over-oxidize the cells, because the iron atoms on the red blood cells can only release the amount of oxygen which the cells can use. When taken orally, stabilized oxygen is non-toxic. There are two kinds of bacteria; aerobic and anaerobic. Aerobic bacteria are the natural flora of the body, and cannot survive without the presence of oxygen. Anaerobic bacteria are the disease, infectious, putrefying and contamination bacteria of the earth, found in water, food, and in the body. However, there are anaerobic bacteria which can live in both oxygen, and non oxygen conditions, but they are not always disease and infectious bacteria."

From the Aerobic 07 literature: "We are always asked, How does oxygen actually kill anaerobic bacteria?" First, these micro-organisms possess an electrical charge. An oxygen molecule is short one electron on it's outer orbit. Build up the oxygen in the blood, and the oxygen molecule will seek out the infectious or putrefying bacteria, and pull the electron away from the micro-organisms. The result, is dead bacterium... We have not found an anaerobic disease that it will not kill... it is virtually tasteless... it is not hydrogen peroxide. It is effective against Salmonella, Cholera, E. Coli, Streptococcus, pseudamonas and Staphylococcus - even against Guardia lamblia"

And, "When there is insufficient oxygen to support the health of a cell, the cell turns to another source of energy, usually sugar fermentation. This is an undesirable source of energy which upsets the metabolism of the cell. It causes the cell to start manufacturing improper chemicals, and soon, a whole group of cells is unhealthy and weak. They loose their natural immune system. they open their doors to the invasion of viruses, for a virus can only develop within a cell. Thus, development of a shortage of oxygen in the blood, could very well be the starting point, for a loss of the immune system and the beginning of feared health problems...."

179

The state of Texas has recently decided the labels for O7 weren't in compliance, so they now ship from Concordia, Missouri, while they make new labels. Apparently they put too much product information on the bottle, and told how to use it, which was called "prescribing without a license". The FDA, however, hasn't objected, and the company has recently applied to have it registered as a food additive (GRAS - Generally regarded as safe). To do this, the Department of Agriculture had to be notified, and since it kills bacteria, it has to be registered as a pesticide with the state, which now says it can't be registered in the state of Texas, since "there is no need for such a product."

Aerobic Life Products was started by Mr. Ed Goodloe, a former large scale farmer and fertilizer manufacturer, who, after years of studying the life processes of plants, and then humans, secured the O7 formula. He's been taking his formula for 18 years, he's 73, and describes himself as: "Perfectly healthy, solid, and I've been assimilating my food properly and building healthy cells in my body. I have more energy than any of these young people who work for me. I keep that colon clean with our colon cleanse, I assimilate my food and then absorb it and those minerals, which come out with the right electrical charge, and build healthy cells in my body."

Stabilized Oxygen, known as Aerobic 07, Aqua Sana, Aqua Pure, and a number of private label brands, is available at $16.50 for a 70ml dropper bottle, which provides 1400 drops. They also have a 1oz. travel size. Also offered, are the previously featured 10 day Colon Cleanse, and various hair, skin care, and juice products, all based on O7. Sold by Aqua Dynamics, 981-OT River Road, Reading, PA 19601 (Aqua Dynamics also sells automatic liquid injectors that put the solution of your choice into water lines). 07 is also available from Aerobic Life Industries, Inc. 3045-OT So. 46th St., Phoenix, AZ 85040. 968-0707

AEROX

After an initial "oral method" hydrogen peroxide cleansing, I switched between taking Aerox (It tastes better than peroxide), and rubbing aloe/hydrogen peroxide into my skin. I used Aerox for about a year and a half. By all subjective evidence, it has boosted my immune system, since many around me got sick sooner or later, and I didn't. I did notice that if I took too many drops of either Aerox, or peroxide, I got a mild "heartburn" a few hours later. So, for me at least, it apparently has a "window" of use, like all our other oxygenation products. 10 to 15 drops of Aerox have no ill effects on me, that I can notice. In fact, just the opposite is true.

Aerox ($NaClO_2$ or Sodium Chlorite), is a "liquid concentrate of electrolytes of oxygen, which are made available to your body, in molecular form, when ingested. Electrolytes are any substances that dissolve in water, and conducts electricity. Its genius, is in formulating a way to have the two most abundant and important electrolytes of body fluid, sodium and chlorine, act as the oxygen carriers. The unique sodium chlorite formulation, stabilizes millions of oxygen molecules in solution with electrons galore. The molecular oxygen is released upon contact with the stomach

180

acid. Aerox helps provide molecular oxygen to your bloodstream. Secondly, it kills anaerobic bacteria and other parasites, on contact, without harming your tissue or friendly aerobic bacteria. There are only 43mg. of salt in 20 drops, a negligible amount. No free chlorine ever escapes in the Aerox formula, according to oxygenation proponent, Tom Valentine, the author of, "Search For Health Newsletter".

CHLORITE IONS

The key to why Aerox works as it does, is the specific "enzyme enhancing" qualities of the chlorite ion. Chemically speaking, the chlorite ion is a molecule of chlorine and oxygen with a strong negative charge. The same molecule with a neutral charge is chlorine dioxide - an even more potent oxidizer; a super effective killer of microbes.

DRINKING AEROX

When you dilute Aerox in water, the highly alkaline pH of the Aerox is rapidly lowered from pH 12-13 to about pH 8.6. This lowering of the pH in water causes the separation of chlorite ions and stabilized oxygen molecules (O_2) from the sodium atoms. Tiny amounts of chlorine dioxide are also released.

This reaction destroys microbes in the water, which makes Aerox is a good thing to have on hand when traveling in foreign countries. When the Aerox water is swallowed, it should encounter stomach acid with a normal pH of 3 to 4. *The reaction created in the stomach environment is even stronger and it generates more molecular oxygen and more chlorite ions and more chlorine dioxide.*

Not only do you have a wealth of energetic dissolved oxygen to be immediately absorbed into the bloodstream, but you have the specific "oxidizers" of chlorite and chlorine dioxide destroying viruses, bacteria and protozoa.

"Aerox has proven effective in killing salmonella, cholera, E. coli, streptococcus, pseudamonas and staphyloccus aureus. Be sure you don't leave home without it when traveling. Yes, now you can drink the water." - APW advertisement.

AEROX MANUFACTURE IS EXACTING

The manufacture of Aerox is an exacting procedure. The manufacturing lab, in the San Francisco Bay area, had a hole blown in it's ceiling once, through an industrial accident, during manufacturing. This is like a rocket fuel, with a lot of oxygen present. Chlorine dioxide gas is not used in it's manufacture. The time-consuming proprietary manufacturing techniques explain why it is more expensive than hydrogen peroxide. Aerox is non-toxic sodium chlorite ($NaClO_2$, $NaClO_4$, NaClOx).

The amount of sodium in the end product is negligible. Cells, particularly leukocytes, use the chlorite to increase the efficiency of peroxidase enzymes. Aerox deactivates phenols. Veterinarians report it inactivates neurotoxins from fungi and moldy foods."
- Biochemist, Dr. James D. Berg, Ph.D., formerly of Stanford.

"It works primarily on the basis of oxidation, apparently being able to supply stimulus to the organisms own physiological response, as well as offering additional oxidative capacity at the cellular level...Where utilized in vivo, it combines with the natural body functions and immune responses to become an effective medication with virtually no toxic or side effects."
- S. Anderson Peoples, MD, Professor of Pharmacology, Univ. CA.

"The reason it works so well is, our bodies are mostly water, and bodily fluids account for most of our body weight. Human blood plasma closely resembles primeval sea water. The red cell carries 99% of our oxygen needs, but the plasma feeds both food and a very important 1% of our oxygen needs to the cells. If the red blood cells are oxygen deficient, it is possible for them to pick up oxygen from the plasma. Cells always get their oxygen from the plasma. Oxygen goes from the red cells, into the plasma, then into the cells. If it is possible to raise the plasma oxygen level, then we can increase the cellular oxygenation level, and provide the red cell a buffer against carbon monoxide! Interstitial fluid, the same as plasma, surrounds every cell in the body. The interior of every cell is also full of water, called "intracellular fluid". Our bodies are about 70% water. 40% of that is inside the cell walls. Ideally, our body water should be teeming with dissolved oxygen. By daily ingestion of Aerox we contribute greatly to maintaining a high cellular fluid oxygen content. It has been shown to kill candida better than orally ingested hydrogen peroxide, and helps improve the white blood cells that make up the immune system. Dr. Peoples has shown that Aerox gets to the cells four times faster than hydrogen peroxide."
- The above from: "Search For Health" the APW Newsbulletin.

A 60 day supply of Aerox, 60 cc's or 1200 drops per bottle, is $21.95. Aerox can be ordered from APW (Associated Partners West), P.O.Box 3048-OT, Iowa City, IA 52244.

USES FOR THESE PRODUCTS

Here are some examples of uses for these products. According to the "Search for Health" newsletter, Aerox can be used as follows:

10 drops in 8 oz. of mountain water can kill Guardia lamblia in 2 1/2 minutes. 20 drops per gallon of water is assumed usually enough to protect clean long term storage water against Coliform disease bacteria.

A drop on a soaked cotton swab can be immediately applied to any insect bite (bees, wasps, mosquitoes, and fire ants).

Put 20 drops in a quart of refrigerated milk, and it will stay fresh for 3 to 4 weeks.

People have used douches and enemas with 30 drops of Aerox per quart, and in colonic machine water. Dr. Koch recommended the use of sodium chloride solutions for bowel cleansing prior to application of his "oxidation starter", and even noted that in the cases where he had limited results, it was due toxin laden colon.

Pets, and house plants, reportedly thrive on it, getting 5 drops per bowl, and race horse owners have used 60 drops per gallon on their horses.

As a food preservative it is said to be unequalled. 10 drops per pint of oil halts rancidity from microbes in oil. Salad bars and vegetables are sprayed or washed with it (60-80 drops/gallon used repeatedly). All meats, fish and poultry remain odorless longer when treated with it. Be careful of putting it directly on your skin, however, the strong alkalinity can burn or scar skin slightly if not diluted first.

WHO'S ON FIRST?

Because you may run into some confusion out there, during the competition of the marketplace, and because your running into it may undermine your confidence in the effectiveness of these products, I'll comment on the stories that are circulating.

From my interviews: the people at Aerobic O7 state that the APW (Aerox) people started out with the O7 formulation, after getting it from them, and continue to use it. On the other side, the APW people state they did sell O7 at first, but now use a different formula for **Aerox**. It appears that, concerning the intertwining history of the formulations, both companies are victims of the passage of the years (possibly up to 50) clouding history, and second hand information. To detail it all would take pages, and is not our subject. I'm not a chemist, but from ancedotal supplier reports, most people using either product claim to have been helped. The evidence continually shows something is occurring, healthwise, so don't let the interplay of their karma get in the way.

The products might be different formulas or not, but, both companies do state, that the strengths are slightly different. As Tom Valentine said, "If you have 98% water, and 2% product, you have O7. If you have 96% water, and 4% product, you have Aerox." Don't be surprised at these concentrations, as both products, for safety, fall within the preferred "window of effectiveness" of each. They are highly alkaline, and not to be used in strong concentrations. Whichever one you may consider, remember, many different people say they've used either one or the other and enjoyed the results.

DIOXYCHLOR (r)

Dioxychlor (r), is different than Aerox or Aerobic 7. ABH or American Biologics, the supplier, is wasting time trying to discredit hydrogen peroxide, and states that Dioxychlor (r) is: an inorganic compound composed of chlorine and two atoms of nascent oxygen, covalently bonded. It is the chemical property of Dioxychlor (r), which makes possible the release of nascent (atomic) oxygen upon decomposition during its action as an oxidizing agent, leaving a non-toxic chlorine residue. In pure form it has a deep red color. Mixed with water, and in a high dilution, it is colorless. When Dioxychlor reacts as an oxidizing agent, the oxygen atom first binds to a single atom (the one being oxidized), and then is dissociated from chlorine. An electron is then given up to chlorine, forming the chloride ion.

Sold only to healthcare professionals, to encourage you to be under the care of a professional, Dioxychlor (r) comes from American Biologics, as a topical gel, homeopathic drops, or as cryogenically purified intravenous infusion material.

From their literature: "Dioxychlor (r), one of a class of inorganic oxidants, has been found useful against the three major classes of infective agents - virus, bacteria, and fungi - and to have tremendous potential use in such refactory conditions as acquired immune deficiency syndrome (AIDS). It is also extremely effective against an impressive array... including demonstrated inhibition of Candida albicans."

Continuing from the sales literature, "Dioxychlor (r) is highly effective at concentrations less than 1 part per million (ppm) that permits it to be used homeopathically. The use of Dioxychlor as a substance dates back to World War 1, when it was used by the Western powers to save the lives of soldiers with infections, particularly gangrene."

The competitors of Dioxychlor (r) question whether it leaves any toxic residue. In their defense, I wonder how something at one part per million is toxic, unless it is given in the wrong dose, or repeatedly.

BIOELECTRICITY

Oxidation is primarily an electric/chemical process. For example, the cerebral-spinal fluid, that serves as the conduit media for our brain and nervous system, is virtually a sea of electrolytes of oxygen, saline oxygen. Ross M. Gwynn, has put forth a theory of "Bioelectrolysis". He states, "Oxygen, ozone, and chlorites are products of electrolysis, and bioelectrolysis suggests that body electricity may generate these helpful oxidants. The greatest concentration of electrolytic fluid is in the cerebral spinal fluid - the media of our magnificent nervous system. There is an, heretofore unreported hyperoxic booster in man, which operates in the bioelectrolysis of cerebral-spinal fluid in the brain, and nerve system, to produce essential life-supporting components, including activated oxygen equivalents."

In simpler allegory, what he is saying is, that the body oxygenation mechanisms (breathing, cell respiration, and production of enzymes, co-enzymes, etc.) are created, by the same methods as electricity making hydrogen and oxygen out of water (electrolysis). It's as if millions of little car batteries are being charged within our bodies. Are the mitochondria the batteries? Some say they are one of our prime links with the invisible sea of energy that we are swimming in.

Further, this electrolysis process is affected by our emotional/mental health. Here's an example: the loss of a loved-one would probably produce a stressful depressive state that lowers our oxygenation processes, and lead to inertia. What's happening, is that our awareness is continually focused upon our emotional pain, and our life forces are being channeled into production of that pain, which diverts our body's electrical resources away from what they're supposed to be doing, charging our batteries, or electrolysis. This produces the stressful beta state, where the brain doesn't put out enough current to even measure. Left unresolved, the lack of bodily electrolysis could lead to hypoxia, malfunction, and then disease. There is an electro-physiological link to being "heart-broken", that is the stuff of psychosomatic illness.

STRESS

"Doctors estimate that 50 to 70 percent of all diseases are at least partially caused by stress" - Prevention Magazine

Another example: I just watched, Martin Sheen (the actor) discuss the heart attack he had, when he was 39, and in the Philippines, filming "Apocalypse Now." He said he realized, finally, that he did it to himself, through not being nice to his family, or others, during those years. Then a specialist was interviewed. He quoted new studies showing how our traditional ideas about "type A", heart-attack-prone people, may only be partly true.

The evidence now shows that **"working hard", or "getting the job done", was not the prime cause of the heart attacks in these cases. What does it, is the negative thoughts these people carry: anger, frustration, blaming others, etc.!** I would explain it this way. We are alive, we eat, we oxidize the food, this produces compounds, chemicals, and electricity that keeps us alive. Since our very thoughts are electrical charges, then, if we indulge the ego, by creating excited, pressured, negative and reversed electrical charges, we negate or confuse the bioelectrical input into our cerebral-spinal electrolysis machines, lowering their output, not producing enough oxygenation, or finally "short-circuiting" them. At this point the ambulance shows up, and we could be pronounced "a very poor oxygenator". We might postulate, therefore, that happy people generally have better bodily oxygen content, oxygenation compounds, lower blood pressure, and better health, than unhappy people. This would follow, because all other factors being equal, a happy person's bodily conduits have the right connections, polarities, and potentials.

GOOD DEEDS

On the healing power of doing good, scientists are finding that good deeds may benefit your immune system. The mind and immune system are intimately linked. Neural pathways connect the brain to the bone marrow and spleen, which produce cells needed to fight infection. Researchers Eileen Rockefeller Growald and Allan Luks, have shown that white blood cells are "exquisitely sensitive to neuropeptides - chemicals produced by the brain."

CURRENT HEALING METHODS

Oriental Acupuncture, Indian Ayurveda, and recent American systems of Polarity Balancing, Rolfing, Chiropractic, Press Point/Reflexology, and Myotherapy, would tie right into this idea. When negative emotion, or injury, or other irritants occur, there is said to be a "blockage" of energy flow, a lessening or stoppage of the life current in one or more areas, organs, or meridian systems.

CHIROPRACTIC

A chiropractor told me that studies have shown that one of the effects of Chiropractic adjustments was to increase oxygenation of the nervous system. If the bioelectrolysis theory is correct, then it would follow that if a site would not "electrolyze" enough, a lowering of oxygenation and it's products would occur in that area or organ. In Acupressure, it is said these sites would collect minute, "crystallized toxins" under the skin, which the trained therapist massages or presses to break them up, restoring the energy flows and health. Those of you familiar with Myotherapy or even the Wilhelm Reich body "armoring" concept (a painful chronic muscular contraction from repressed emotion), will notice the similarities.

I would like to point out, that I found much of this interwoven throughout the world's ancient spiritual teachings, having been passed down for centuries. It's just that it's not readily available to someone without an open mind, or who's not willing to do a lot of investigation out of the mainstream.

OTHER ELECTRON TRANSPORT PRODUCTS

This isn't strictly an oxygenation subject, but it's closely related, since oxygenation ultimately ends up being a booster of the electron transporting systems at the atomic cell level. Two such reported boost enhancers are: "Cancell" and "Golden Wonder" both provided by the Herb and Mineral Research Labs, Inc., 3704-OT Chestnut Ave., Newport News, VA 23607.

CANCELL AND GOLDEN WONDER

From their admittedly technical literature: "Cancell is a new chemical combination which is effective in the treatment of neoplasms, collagen diseases, and many other "protein" diseases...it is a further object of Cancell (to) induce lysis of the aberrant structures.. (by effecting a shift in energy structures and) reducing the rate of ATP supply while maintaining or increasing, the rate of high energy (ee-H+)- supply". They supplied me with a document suggesting Cancell helped Lukemia victims. Their other product, "Golden Wonder", contains crystalline gold. Rubbed into the skin, it reportedly seems to beneficially restore some of the cell and muscular electrical balance, and greatly lessen the pain of some arthritis, muscular, and other, conditions. A friend of mine used it on a chronically painful shoulder, with benefit.

GOLD INJECTIONS

The above products immediately remind me of "gold injections". If you know anyone who has arthritis, then you probably know about one of the current medical treatments, injecting a gold solution into a arthritis patient, to eliminate pain. The gold, probably, is restoring the body electrical system function, by introducing a pathway creating a higher energy of electron transport. The only problem with the injection method, is that it has to be monitored closely for the possibility of dangerous toxicity, since we aren't built to eat metal, only to use it as an organically bound trace mineral.

GOLD USE BY EGYPTIANS

Gold may not be a natural food, but it is a great electrical conductor. The connector plugs on the back of "high end" stereos are plated with it, guaranteeing perfect electrical conductivity. In Boston, the Museum of Fine Arts has an Egyptian section that displays (in glass cases) ancient Egyptian "Vril" sticks. Vril sticks are short hollow metal tubes that were held in the hand of temple priests who were schooled in the secret teachings. These intricately detailed tubes are composed of a secret mixture of quartz, gold and silver, called "electrinium".

The museum doesn't say what they were used for, but a study of the ancient literature reveals claims that initiates - who had trained their consciousnesses sufficiently - used them by holding the hollow tubes out in their hands and creating a psionic vortex that focused and channeled their higher energies through the tubes. With the use of these tubes, they were said to be capable of healing, levitation, and other phenomena. The current crowd enamored with the use of crystals, also claims that gold amplifies auric emanations.

From this information, we can suspect that gold has very important higher electrical properties, and possible further healing applications that we aren't aware of. It seems to me that all this medical and ancedotal information is connected, and deserves further research.

PEOPLE AND PLACES USING OXYGENATION

U.S. DOCTORS USING H2O2 THERAPY

THERE ARE DOCTORS WHO CONSIDER H2O2 LEGAL TO ADMINISTER IN THE US, AS IT IS ONLY A NATURALLY OCCURRING BODILY SUBSTANCE. WRITE TO IBOM FOR INFORMATION AND REFERRALS. Hopefully, the FDA will agree if they ever have to rule on it. IBOM, Ozone & Peroxide Referrals, P.O. Box 13205-OT, Oklahoma City, OK 73113, phone 405/478-4266.

DOCTORS AND CLINICS USING H2O2 AND OZONE

NOTE: The printing of this information, is to allow any doctors wishing to do further research to look up these people and places. I **am not advertising for, or referring you** (or anyone else) **to these places!** I have never been to any of them, I don't know for sure what they do there, and I am not medically qualified to judge either the clinics, or people to whom I refer. In the U.S., it is illegal to use ozone at present, so the doctors here use hydrogen peroxide. In Germany it is illegal to use hydrogen peroxide, but ozone use has been legal for over 30 years.

MEXICO & GERMANY

GERSON INSTITUTE CLINICS c/o POB 430-OT, Bonita, CA, 92002. Charlotte Gerson teaches only a whole systems approach to health.

DONSBACH ROSARITA BEACH CLINIC One of this book's main speaker's organizations. C/O 323-OT E. San Ysidro Blvd, San Ysidro, CA, 92073 619/428-8585

KELLNER CLINIC Baden Weiler, Federal Republic of Germany. An elegant hotel/resort/clinic/retreat in the Black Forest. Located on the edge of Switzerland. They've been treating people for 25 years, with ozone, and other modalities, that are available only outside of the U.S.. In 1987 it cost approximately $3,000 to stay there and be treated for a few weeks.

ROSARITA BEACH CLINIC Located in Mexico, with a U.S. Office, is run by Dr. Gary Young who does hydrogen peroxide infusions. 706/689-4465 or 619/426-2002.

GUADALAJARA MEDICAL SCHOOL The Guadalajara Medical School, Mexico's largest, is about to test bio-oxidative therapies, and possibly incorporate them into their curriculum.

DR. HEINZ KONRAD M.D. of Sao Paulo, Brazil, reports an 85% success rate in treating herpes with ozone.

DR. S. RILLING, of Stuttgart, is with Arztlich Gesellschaft fur Ozontherapie, and Dr. Renate Viebahn, of Iffezheim, is with JrJ Hansler GmbH. Probably two of the most famous and knowledgeable ozone proponents, they have authored many ozone writings, conducted seminars, and delivered many addresses on ozone usage.

DR. HORST KIEF, Specialist in Ozontherapy. In the Munich area of West Germany, he is said to be using ozone to completely eliminate the AIDS virus in it's victims by ozonation.

DR. VARO, Duseldorf, Germany. One of the best known ozone therapists. An elder experienced gentleman.

ALEXANDER PREUSS Featured in this book as claiming successful AIDS treatments. D-700 Stuttgart 1 (West) Bebel Strasse 29, Federal Republic of Germany.

USA

INTERNATIONAL BIO-OXIDATIVE MEDICINE FOUNDATION P.O. Box 61767-OT, Dallas/Ft. Worth, TX 75261. They refer anyone to the closest MD currently using intravenous hydrogen peroxide in the US.

MEDIZONE 2B-OT, E. 54th St., New York, NY 10022. Holds US patent on ozonation of mammalian blood. Completing lab studies, and working toward FDA approval for human testing and treatment with ozone in the US. Medizone is also setting up operations in Europe and Asia.

DR. CHRISTIAN BERNARD, the famous heart transplant surgeon, said in March 1986 that he takes hydrogen peroxide himself, to reduce arthritis and aging. Dr. C. Bernard, Oklahoma Heart Center, 3300 Northwest Expressway, Oklahoma City, OK, 73112.

DR. KURT DONSBACH at the Bio Genesis Institute in Rosarita Beach, Baja, Mexico, (above) has pointed out that no U.S. clinic or institution has ever tested intravenous H_2O_2 as a treatment for cancer, so any claim that it is not effective, is not based on clinical trial, but speculation.

DR. CHARLES FARR, author of "The Therapeutic Use of Intravenous Hydrogen Peroxide", directs The International Bio-oxidative Medicine Foundation, and publishes the IBOM Newsletter, which physicians use as a reference in refining the H_2O_2 infusion process. he has reported that H_2O_2: "kills bacteria, protozoa, yeast, and virus, has oxidized lipids from arterial walls, increases oxygen tension intracellularly, stimulates oxidative enzymes, returns elasticity to arterial walls, dilates coronary vessels and regulates membrane transport" IBOM #2. IBOM POB 61767-OT, Dallas, TX, 75261. Dr. Farr 11330-OT North May Ave., Oklahoma City, OK 73120

DR. A. J. McDONALD, P.O.Box 775-OT, Lodi, CA, 95240. Familiar with and sells food grade hydrogen peroxide.

DR. GENE MEYER Dr. Meyer tried using the German Biozone machine, with Mr. Butch McCabe in Mexicali. He tried many different ozonation applications, including ozonating ice in the preparation of seafood. Dr. Meyer used the University of Minnesota's database, and found thousands of articles on ozone, and has 5,000 articles on hydrogen peroxide.

He told me: not all free radicals are bad, oxygen is one of the good ones. Presently using a blood microscopy machine, wet blood, and dark field microscopy to see what happens when you use ozone. Using "Micron" $30,000 microscope, computers, and a 20 minute lag time. They use 42 micrograms per cc, running 200 cc's three times. He considers this a lot, and warns against using too much, which will decrease the patient's immunity. Each person is a little different.

He tried using ozone on AIDS patients in Mexico. They were late-stage victims, and all died anyway. He has now decided to not use the, "only one treatment", therapy technique. This would agree with the U.S. Medizone and German methods of repeated applications. Dr. Gene Meyer, Biochemist, D.D.S. 9725-OT E. Flower St. Bellflower, CA 90706

CLYMER HEALTH CLINIC, uses a whole systems approach to health, RD #3-OT, Quakertown, PA 18951

PROMINENT OXYGENATION LAY PEOPLE

REVEREND RICHARD R. WILLHELM, we started this book with him, he's extremely knowledgeable, having studied with Dr. Rosenow at Mayo years ago. He has made it his calling to spread the word about hydrogen peroxide. 6600-OT Trail Blvd., N. Naples, FL 33940.

WALTER GROTZ, the most active proponent, and knowledgeable resource, of hydrogen peroxide's benefits, history, and effects. He offers tapes, literature, and a newsletter. He also did a library computer search, and found 4,000 peer-reviewed medical articles, on the application of hydrogen peroxide. If you would like the names and addresses (and phone numbers) of people who claim to have been helped by the use of the hydrogen peroxide program, please write ECHO, next listing.

E.C.H.O. (Educational Concerns for Hydrogen and Oxygen). Dept. OT, P.O.B. 126, Delano, MN 55328. ECHO's good work is donation sponsored, so when you ask for anything, be sure to take care of them.

TOM VALENTINE and his family publish "Search For Health" an oxygenation newsletter promoting the APW line of products. APW, P.O. Box 3048-OT, Iowa City, IA 52244.

WAVES FOREST "Cancer growths contract and disappear when oxygen saturation is sufficiently increased in the fluids surrounding them, since they are anaerobic." Great source for many of this books subjects. Waves and I were working along parallel lines on different coasts. He publishes a newsletter, "Now What?" P.O. Box 768-OT, Monterey, CA, 93942, USA. By Waves Forest, issue 1, Fall of 87.

HECTOR DELAFUENTE, Homeopathic Doctor and Ph.D. in Natural Science, was a friend and assistant of Dr. Koch. P.O. Box 711, San Carlos, CA 94070.

ZANE BARANOWSKI author and Antioxidant enzyme product distributor. Writes about necessity of antioxidants in the oxygenation process. 597-OT Glenwood Cutoff, Scotts Valley, CA 95006.

ED MCCABE The author of "OXYGEN THERAPIES, A NEW WAY OF APPROACHING DISEASE." He wrote the first book to examine, in detail, all known historical and modern oxygenation methods, and the specialists and proponents associated with them. Includes a thorough review of modern products and sources as well. Ed McCabe, c/o Energy Publications, 99-RD #1, Morrisville, NY 13408.

INTERNATIONAL OXIDATION INSTITUTE, ASMM recently changed it's name to INTERNATIONAL INSTITUTE FOR OXYGEN THERAPIES. This group headed by Dr. George Freibott, holds the Blass Homozone patents, and sells a number of Dr. Koch's books. They also have ozone articles, past and current IOI (International Oxidation Institute) newsletters and bulletins, reprints of papers by F.M. Eugene Blass, ND, DC., and other oxygenation items and resources. They will soon have a computer bulletin board system.

From their literature: "Up until the present, there have been virtually NO outlets for information on the historical uses, and administration of the specialized oxidation therapies available in the world today. There is now a group willing to issue specialized reports, leaflets and information on these substances. This is being done strictly as an educational service to the public and healing arts alike. Technical data is available upon request." A subscription is $10 per year. The International Institute For Oxygen Therapies, Inc. (IIOT) P.O. Box 1360-OT, Priest River, ID 83856

Betsy Russell-Manning editor of "Candida, Silver (mercury) Fillings and the Immune System", 1985. Greensward Press, P.O. Box 99472-OT, San Francisco, CA 94109. An excellent collection of references, includes a chapter on hydrogen peroxide.

DR. SCOTT J. GREGORY, M.S., Ph.D., from Santa Monica, CA, works with BIANCA LEONARDO Ph.D., and has a number of AIDS patients taking Hydrogen Peroxide, as part of the "Gregory Method" for years, and only one died. He wrote the book "Conquering AIDS". His new book is called "They Conquered AIDS". Dr. Scott Gregory, P.O.B. 1222-OT Santa Monica, CA 90406.

CHARLES MARCHAND Charles Marchand was a prolific writer. Between 1880 and 1904 he authored 18 H_2O_2 books. For example, he had a 360 page book he wrote on hydrogen peroxide in 1904. More than half the book was reproductions of published medical articles of the times on hydrogen peroxide. They were treating syphilis, gonorrhea, cancer, hay fever, cystitis, and others. We are trying to find any of his materials, he was from France and lived in NYC. He was probably published in the New York Journal of Medicine. If you have, or know of, a source of any of his books, please write me.

A. J. CULLINANE, since the 60's has been advocating the scientific use of saline hydrogen peroxide to raise the blood pH up to normal (6.7 to 7) or above, and thereby "eradicating all disease", since "a virus will only survive and proliferate below pH 7." Some of this theory is disputed by others. The above referenced IIOT has copies of his work: "The Theory of Natural Immunity By Reference To The Saline Oxygen Level Of The Blood And Plasma - The Effect Of The pH Value".

BSRF - Borderland Science Research Foundation Where I first got the word about oxygenation. Articles and reprints on ozone, Koch, MWO, Royal Rife, Merlin, etc. Subscription. P.O. Box 429-OT Garberville, CA 95440

NUTRITIONAL RESEARCH, Information on Rife Microscopes. P.O. Box 652-OT, Milwaukee, Wisconsin, 53201

CANCER BOOK HOUSE full line of alternative therapies by Koch, etc. 2043-OT N. Berendo, Los Angeles, CA 90027.

Super Science, PO Box 392-OT, Dayton, OH, 45409, MWO articles.

OUR PLANET FINDS IT HARDER TO BREATHE

To feed our civilization's industrial requirements; like making fast food, and the bags and containers to carry it in, thousands and thousands of forest acres are being cut down daily. These are mostly the huge Central American tropical rain forests. All the trees, in 55 square feet of rain forest, must be cut down, and turned into grazing land, to provide you with 1/4 pound of beef. 138 million pounds of beef were imported from Central America in 1987. This growing consumption required 696,969 square acres, or, 1,089 square miles of grazing land. People who watched it happen, say that the U.S.'s once enormous green forests, in the West, are all mostly gone now. They say you could watch the changes from commercial airplane flights, and that the loggers always leave a strip of trees on the highway, so you won't notice. I saw this throughout the state of Georgia. Trees put oxygen into our atmosphere. No trees, no oxygen.

The increasing waste products from our civilization are finding their way to the oceans, or being dumped there. Besides poisoning the whales, dolphins, fish, shrimp, and clams, this kills marine vegetation that puts oxygen into our atmosphere. No marine vegetation, no oxygen.

The front page of the Canadian newspapers ran a story recently, explaining that scientists had analyzed the content of some gas bubbles that were trapped in prehistoric substances. They concluded, that there was twice as much oxygen in the atmosphere back then.

Dr. Otto Warburg said, that if you deprive a cell 60% of it's oxygen, it will turn cancerous. Do you live in a city, or work in an environment where the oxygen content is down to 10%? Is it any wonder, that there is such an epidemic of chronic degenerative disease, that 1/3 of our population suffers from something?

Profits are sometimes hard to come by, because competition is tough. Along the way, it's sometimes easy to go for the "quick" solutions while ignoring the environment. Let's have a balance between the present and long term needs of all of us, and our children, and the immediate needs of the few.

THE NEW WORLD PHYSICS

Here's a new viewpoint for your analysis, concerning our ozone layer problems. We have heard about the danger to our ozone layer from flourocarbons. According to Lloyd Zirbes, Ph.D., what most of us aren't aware of, is that there is an unrecognized danger - a new class of tiny particles. This new class of particles is so small that they are not being studied by the main body of our scientists. Mr. Zirbes states that these super small "diverted" or "fine" particles are emitted from any use of electrical transformation and transmission, all radio and TV transmissions, and any nuclear material.

Since 1900 (when we started applying the electron theory), our planet core has begun heating up. We now have severe droughts, increasing yearly. The reason we have a planetary heat buildup, is simple. These small, "emitted particles" are collecting in our upper atmosphere, and natural magnetic fields, and are being carried by them, back through the earth's core. This is occurring at an increasing density and rate. As they pass through the core, they compress, and give up heat. We haven't studied them, because, in general, our scientists don't have the instrumentation able to go down to that small a range and measure them. Mr. Zirbes has done tests, and worked out all the math to identify them.

Mr. Zirbes has made the tests and discoveries necessary, to develop a body of knowledge explaining these phenomenon. He calls it: "The New World Physics". In this work, he proves, that in a gravitational field, (in other words, anywhere, on any planet) all falling bodies do not fall at the same rate. What everyone was taught about gravity, in school, is incorrect. Worse yet, present day physics is based upon Einstein, who based his work on Newton, who based his work on Galileo - Galileo's hypothetical tests on falling bodies from the leaning tower of Pisa. Galileo never dropped anything off the tower of Pisa! He sat home and imagined what would happen, if he dropped objects off the tower. Even if he had done the tests, the tower is only 64 feet tall, and tests from such a short height wouldn't show any acceleration differences.

Mr. Zirbes, in 1961, performed tests on falling bodies using a 2,000 foot mineshaft, and proved that bodies do not fall at the same rate. He proved that $E=MC^2$ is incorrect. He invites anyone who doubts this, to spend years of their lives dropping things down mineshafts, as he has. Mr. Zirbes states that because our whole industry is based upon a science developed under these errors, our entire planet is in mortal danger. The danger, is from global heating, and, in danger from electrical storms. This will lead to further droughts, which will produce famines. All this will eventually produce climatic disasters. He concludes, that our only hope lies in shifting, from an electron science based economy, to a gravity science based economy. This will only be possible with the cooperation of everyone on the planet, because there is only a short time left, in which we will be able to effect positive changes. He further says, the rate of change is increasing geometrically. Mr. Zirbes has fully documented his findings of the last 30 years.

He explains these tiny particles, and the danger to our ozone, thusly (paraphrased): To give you an idea of the problem of measuring these tiny diverted particles, please imagine the super small size of an electron. Now, in your mind, expand that electron tremendously, up to the size of the huge planet Jupiter. Now imagine one of the tiny moons that orbits Jupiter... That's how small these diverted or fine particles are, compared to an electron, roughly 1/80th the size.

The closest thing to these diverted particles that our scientists have come up with, are the new, speculative, so called, "no mass" particles. Trouble is, they do have mass! These particles are so energetic and so small, that they pass right through any containment walls or insulation, and are combining with the earth's magnetic fields at an ever increasing geometric rate.

Collecting in the upper atmosphere, these particles are combining with, and altering, the chemical makeup of our planetary oxygen and other chemicals, and even creating strange new combinations and heat. This is the answer to two questions that the international scientists are pondering: the billions of tons of carbon that is "missing" from the carbon cycle, and the need to find the mysterious source of the increasing levels of methane and nitrous oxide. Do you remember in a previous chapter I showed you how ozone and nitrogen, under heat, in a reaction, formed nitric acid? Mr. Zirbes claims this is what is happening in our upper atmosphere.

These reactions in our upper atmosphere are also binding up our oxygen, rendering it unable to react, and therefore, unable to be turned into ozone by the sun. Thus, we are losing our ozone supply. As you saw earlier, ultraviolet light striking oxygen is the mechanism used to produce ozone in medical ozone generators.

"**Normally, oxygen, O_2, absorbs ultraviolet radiation, which sets off a chemical reaction, which produces ozone.** If oxygen were not so isotopic, it would not be able to accept this ultraviolet radiation. Normal, highly isotopic oxygen is a natural "magnet" to these fission released, diverted fine particles, which are drawn to, and attempt to, assimilate with the normal oxygen. As more and more fine particles assimilate with the oxygen atoms, within the O2 molecule, these atoms become heavier, less isotopic, and finally radioactive, as they become a negative plasma. Without their isotopic quality, the oxygen molecules cannot absorb ultraviolet radiation from the sun, and therefore cannot produce ozone. Ultraviolet radiation which is not absorbed will find its way to the earth and life forms below."
- From "Fine Particles - A Test" L. Zirbes, Ph.D.

This means, that when the sun strikes the atmosphere, it does not produce enough life sustaining ozone - which should be reacting with only natural elements, breaking down pollutants, and putting oxygen into the food chain. Not enough ozone (and hydrogen peroxide) is falling to earth in rain and snow, resulting in increasingly less re-oxygenation of the planet. These fine, diverted particles are amassing, due to magnetic repulsion and attraction, and causing holes in the ozone. The news media's favorite scapegoat, the CFC's - refrigerant gasses - have little to do with it. There are now holes in our ozone at <u>both</u> poles, as well as other places around our planet. The ozone layer is actually starting to resemble swiss cheese.

OK, at this point you may not believe it, so, here's your own experiment, from the above paper. Go to the hardware store, and get a small cylinder of oxygen, sold for homeowner torches. Get permission to place it as close as you can, but <u>outside</u> of the lead, steel, and concrete containment structure of a fission reactor. Place it high up, downwind, and in a shaded spot. Be sure no one tampers with it. Leave it there for a few weeks. Then, remove it, and take it to a commercial ozone gas producer or manufacturer. Have him try and turn the oxygen gas in the exposed cylinder into ozone. There will be great difficulty in achieving a complete conversion to ozone. If the cylinder was left exposed long enough, none of the oxygen will combine into ozone. Just like in the atmosphere, the oxygen becomes saturated with diverted fine particles, and can no longer change. An alternative test, would be to (cautiously) float oxygen balloons near high voltage lines, radio towers, a large transformer, or a radar installation. Analyze the gas before and after the test period. Analysis, after the test, will show: H, H_2, H_3, H_2O, ClO, He, F, Be, B, Li, and a number of strange chemical combinations in the balloon gas that weren't there before. Zirbes Enterprises, Rte. 1, Box 206-OT, Foreston, MN 56330.

Because of the increasing ozone depletion factor, many scientists are privately betting that we might not have a planet that can support life for long. The oxygen levels are dropping, and droughts and electrical storms might continue to increase. Some speculate the only answer is to leave here and colonize another planet. Let's not give up on this planet, yet. We must use our creativity to change our policies, and consciousness, here, now. Otherwise, when we go into space, we'll just bring our problems with us, "infecting" someplace else, and have to learn the same lessons there.

Let's apply our technology and research efforts to re-oxygenating and re-ozonating this world, and our bodies. It is not impossible, or too late. Assuming that it is, is to ignore our creativity, and we'll seal our fate. We have to overcome the reactive human mind which, in a reflex action, tends to give up, or flee, when faced with a difficult challenge.

The same principals will apply to the "living organism earth", as to when we re-oxygenate our bodies for health. Oxygen and ozone are the substances that nature uses to de-pollute the planet. We need to stop polluting, and start developing and using new sciences, sciences that incorporate efficient uses of our

195

resources. We need to find new ways to re-oxygenate our bodies and our environment. Then, all we have to do, is insure that no future mistakes are incorporated into our ways of life. We can do this.

PRIMARY DISEASE CAUSE?

CALL TO INVESTIGATION
Medical science has always looked for the primary physical cause of all diseases. Poor oxygenation, and improper electron transport at the cellular level, is almost certainly one of the basic "It's". But the concept is so simple, that some professionals, who haven't done the research, have a hard time believing it. They might be getting so involved in details, or so involved in the defense of cherished ideals, that they aren't open to new input, or noticing the big picture.

Our most abundant and essential element is oxygen. Remember, of all the elements the body needs, only oxygen is in such constant demand that its absence brings death in minutes.

In the face of thousands of people, now claiming they have been healed (partially, or completely), of "incurable" disease, by oxygenation methods using hydrogen peroxide, ozone, etc., we definitely need, an all-out effort to conduct scientific case studies. Then we can provide documentation to convert the final skeptics. If you join in this effort, you will definitely be helping humanity.

ALTERNATIVE DISCIPLINES

From here on, because many in this enlightening age will wonder how their favorite disciplines, theories, or beliefs, fit into our oxygenation subject, I'll take the liberty of discussing some alternative subjects. Many say these alter life towards a more positive expression.

MACROBIOTICS

The Macrobiotic teachers like Michio Kushi, have shown that: when our body/machines have all the physical and mental/emotional elements needed for chemical reactions, in the proper amounts and configurations, they usually heal themselves. Many attribute this to our Divine origins, some to the power of DNA. A study of Macrobiotics reveals a concentration on eating fresh, whole foods. Fresh, whole foods are full of oxygen, and hydrogen peroxide, both taken up by plants from rainwater, and the photosynthesis process.

Many people have documented cases, of being rid of cancer and other diseases, by following a true Macrobiotic diet. I once met a middle-aged woman, who stated she was so full of various diseases, that she went from a "walker", to not being able to sit up, or lie down, or stand. She reached the point of being propped up in bed all the time. After having every available medical treatment her doctors could think of, she went on a Macrobiotic diet. When I met her, she was smiling and walking around, and delivering the lecture with ease.

Having attended some classes on Macrobiotics, I believe that a correct Macrobiotic diet will supply everything needed by a normal body to produce the correct peroxide, and other, reactions in the immune system, and ward off disease. A Macrobiotic lifestyle takes time to prepare daily. The Kushi Foundation has further information Macrobiotics, and holds retreats and seminars in Becket, MA. Kushi Foundation, P.O.B. 1100-OT, 17 Station St., Brookline, MA 02147. Contact them for further information, including books and videos.

FOOD VITALITY CHART

ANGSTROM WAVELENGTH	FRUIT	RAW VEGETABLES	COOKED VEGETABLES	GRAINS	OILS	ANIMAL PRODUCTS	MISC.
9000	ALL FRESHLY PICKED FRUIT	FRESH VEGETABLES, CARROT TOMATO, LEEK ONION BEAN, MUSHROOM RADISH, FRESH SALAD, WINTER CARROT	FRESH INGREDIENT SOUPS, BAKED POTATO, BRAISED VEG	ROLLED OATS, WHOLE WHEAT, SELMOLINA, SPROUTS	FRESH NUTS, BLACK OLIVES, ALMONDS, OLIVE OIL, NUT OILS, COCONUTS	JUST SMOKED, FRESH HAM, FRESH SEA FISH, RAW SHELL FISH, FRESHLY CHURNED BUTTER	CRUDE CANE SUGAR, FRESH SEA SALT, SUPERIOR HONEYS, HERB TEAS
8500	FRESH FRUIT JUICE		BRAISED CABBAGE		DRIED NUTS, GREEN OLIVES		
7500	DRIED FIG, DATE		BOILED PEAS	BUCKWHEAT FLOUR			
6500	HUMAN BODY LEVEL		BOILED POTATOES (WITH SKIN)	WHOLE WHEAT PASTRIES	PEANUT OIL	FRESH MILK	AGING HONEY
5000	DEHYDRATED FRUIT		BOILED ARTICHOKE, COLD POTATO	TAPIOCA, SEMOLINA		FRESH EGG, FRESHWATER FISH	NATURAL WINE, DRIED HERBS
4000	COOKED FRUIT COMPOTE	DEHYDRATED VEGETABLES	MASHED POTATO (NO SKIN)		PUMPKIN SEED OIL	RAW MEAT	SUPERIOR WHITE WINE
3000	GREEN OR OVER RIPE FRUIT	RAW ARTICHOKE, DEHYDRATED VEG. SOUP	OVERCOOKED VEGETABLES	WHITE FLOUR		1 MO.+ EGGS	ORDINARY RED WINE
2000	DECAYING FRUIT	RAW POTATO		WHITE BREAD	STALE OIL		
1000		WITHERING VEG.		5-6 MO. OLD FLOUR		ORDINARY COOKED MEATS	ROCK SALT
0	ROTTING FRUIT, CANNED FRUIT, PASTURIZED JUICE	CANNED	CANNED	6+ MO. OLD FLOUR	MARGARINE, OLD FISH, REFINED OIL	PASTEURIZED MILK- BUTTER, FERMENT. CHEESE, POWDERED EGGS	REFINED WHITE SUGAR, COFFEE, ALCOHOL, TEA, CHOCOLATES

AUTHOR'S NOTE: I HAVE NOTICED THAT WHEN I EAT FOODS NEAR THE TOP OF THIS CHART, I FEEL HEALTHIER. I WOULD ASSUME THEY CONTRIBUTE TO MORE OXYGENATION OF THE BODY, ALTHOUGH I HAVE NOT FOUND A STUDY SHOWING THIS YET. IT'S BEEN IN MY FILES FOR YEARS, I DON'T KNOW WHO THE AUTHOR IS. I ALWAYS KNEW I'D SHOW IT TO SOMEONE, SO HERE IT IS. OUR THANKS TO THE UNKNOWN AUTHOR.

BIOLOGICAL TRANSMUTATION OF ELEMENTS

There are people saying that it is possible, by raising the oxygen level and pH of a diseased cell's environment, to return it to normal. I consider this possibly very important

I once discovered a little book printed by Kushi's Macrobiotic teacher, George Ohsawa, who studied at the Sorbonne and the Pasteur Institute, in Paris. Ohsawa's Macrobiotic Foundation is at 1544 Oak St., Oroville, CA 95965. In it, he documents the little known work of Mr. L. Kervran and Prof. Baranger of the Institut Polytechnique, in Paris. They document 13 years of work, proving that elements can transmute to other elements in the biological body! They reported that sodium becomes potassium, which becomes calcium. Sodium becomes magnesium, etc. Their work was not understood, according to them, due to linear, instead of logarithmic "Golden Ratio" spiral thinking, on the part of critics.

The book cites the creation of high carbon steel that won't rust, by fusing nonmetallic carbon, between two electrodes. Supposedly, there is a high carbon steel pole standing in the earth, near Delhi, India, which has not rusted in thousands of years. I do not know their methods, if anyone has tried to repeat these experiments, or if this is true. For another example, I also heard that Dr. A. Puharich has stated that, in France, grain was specially raised on totally silicon soil, in other words, no calcium, and fed to chickens. The chickens were not fed any calcium, but were able to transform silicon into calcium in their bodies. Also, in another study, brewers yeast, raised in stainless steel tanks (stainless steel is only nickel and iron), was able to take the nickel out of the stainless steel, and produce chromium. If true, it seems that Nature can transmute elements.

My studies continually prove that there is much more to life than we presently acknowledge. These experiments should be replicated by someone, and be open to discussion at all times. There is room for us all, on the palette of life.

So, while we're out on the cutting edge of consciousness, and thinking it just might be possible for elements to transmute, let's look at the work of Royal R. Rife...

ROYAL R. RIFE

A scientist and biologist. His work ties into the treatment of cancer, etc., so it's presented as a possible explanation, as to why ozone and H_2O_2 are effective at the micro cellular level.

As an inventor, Mr. Rife worked with the upper frequencies of light, and their harmonics. The reader is reminded, that light, and everything else, is a collection of frequencies. Light and sound are only separate octaves of frequencies, different harmonics of energy. Our ears sense (hear) within a certain range, and our eyes sense (see) within another, and our television picks up another (radio frequencies), and converts it into a range we can see and hear easily.

INVENTS SUPER MICROSCOPES

Mr. Rife, invented Rife Microscopes, that had much greater range than those commonly used today, and had the advantage of not changing the cells or microbes being observed. His Rife microscopes were based upon light, not electrons. His major discovery, was that by applying certain frequencies to a cancer cell, he could over time, change it back to a normal cell, or vice versa! Some are proposing we do this, to AIDS viruses, with pulsed red laser light. Rife wrote many papers on his work.

MICROBES EXIST BEYOND OUR VISUAL RANGE

Using the magnified output of light as it splits up, and passes through quartz prisms, he discovered (by seeing them at work), that there were microorganisms existing just beyond our limited eyesight range. He discovered them living in the ultraviolet, and infrared frequency ranges, and that they were causing many "unknown cause" diseases.

He took two frequencies, "A" and "B", and combined them. As in music, this combination produced two other new harmonic frequencies, one their additive, (A+B), and one their subtractive, (A-B). He worked with the differences between the two, their lower harmonics.

In other words, the ultraviolet range of light, is much larger than the one octave of normal light we use for vision. Rife focused two invisible ultraviolet lights on a specimen, at the same time, and produced a light that was the difference between them, and visible.

Because of this illumination, the microorganisms that had no visible colors in our limited normal visible range, could be seen in their natural living state, without stains.

TRADITIONAL MICROSCOPES FUZZY

In traditional high power microscopes, light reflected off the specimen passes up through the barrel of the scope. It doesn't stay in parallel rays, but crosses, and then spreads out again. This makes the image fuzzy at high magnifications.

ELECTRON MICROSCOPES KILL SPECIMENS

Also, stains, or electrons, from electron microscopes kill what we're looking at, so we never get to truly see it. In contrast, Rife Microscopes use prisms, to spread the light into parallel rays going up the tube, before it crosses. Stacked up, these quartz prisms keep the lightrays parallel. Much clearer and more highly magnified images result. More technical details on the microscopes can be obtained from the Lee Foundation for Nutritional Research, P.O.B. 652, Milwaukee, Wisconsin, 53201 - reprint #47 "The Rife Microscopes, or Facts and Their Fate".

MAKES ULTRAVIOLET MICROBES VISIBLE

He found that, by changing the combinations of the two light-rays focused on a specimen, he could choose (tune to) any portion of the ultraviolet, and make it visible. He also discovered that disease cells and microbes each have their own frequencies. Therefore, he was able to tune into (make visible) any particular microbe. He found that each type of microbe had it's own life frequency emitting range, or color, which was always the same.

CELL VIRUSES MUTATE WITH ENVIRONMENTAL CHANGES

He reported in his extensive works, that he discovered viruses for cancer and polio this way. Because he didn't have to kill them to see them, he could experiment on them. He changed the solution that the cancer viruses were trapped in slightly (four parts per million), and he was amazed to see them, in time, turn into larger viruses. Another change and they turned into single cells. With more solution changes, the cells became fungi, then aerobic bacteria!

OXYGENATION COULD PREVENT OR REVERSE MUTATIONS?

This, dear reader, (I've always wanted to use that phrase) brings us home again, to "How does the ozone, or peroxide, or free radical oxygen rid us of diseases like cancer?" Do you remember Dr. Otto Warburg, twice Nobel Prize Laureate, who proved that cancer cells live by fermentation? They are anaerobic, they only exist if there's little oxygen around. So, perhaps cellular oxygenation, besides providing outright destruction of pathogens, changes the cell solutions enough, to transform an area of disease production back to normal, just like Rife found out. Maybe anaerobic, "fermentation type" diseased cells, can turn into aerobic bacteria, or even back to normal cells. This is what Rife maintained, that slight changes in body tissue could change one microorganism into another, in the same group. There would seem to be a lot of research that needs to be done in these areas.

I brought these stories out to stimulate discussion, I'm not a doctor or a chemist, and this is not my theory, although it is logical to me. I'll explain: an organism, large or small, has a very strong survival factor programmed into it. It will do anything to live, even adapt to very different conditions. Change a person's environment, they adapt to the new one, or perish. This is life. So, if we apply this to Rife's work, then the environment we create in our own bodies is unique. It's a combination of exactly what we eat, what we think, what we do, how we feel, and what happens to us. These factors all combine into a specific environmental range at the cellular level. Our specific, self-created range, is only hospitable to certain shapes, sizes, and types of organisms. Any cells within it, must adapt or perish.

This is why it is so important how you live, because it determines your cellular environments, and therefore, what types of organisms set up housekeeping in you. Good and bad alike. It's up to you, it always has been.

BSRF has a video on Rife's work, and phamplets too. Borderland Sciences Research Foundation, Inc. P.O. Box 429-OT Garberville, CA 95440-0429

GETTING MORE OXYGEN IN YOUR LUNGS

EXERCISE AND RUNNING

The NIH (National Institute of Health), did a five year study at Stanford University School of Medicine. They compared 498 long distance runners, to 365 average people, and found, that the deep breathing (oxygenating) runners: developed the usual age related disabilities at a slower rate, had better cardiovascular (heart) conditions, and weighed less. They went to see a doctor only one third as many times as the average person, and had better attendance records at work. When I explained this subject to a friend who studies yoga, she exclaimed, "That's why all the yogis, who practice alternate nostril breathing for two hours every morning, don't get sick!"

If you're athletic, you will be very interested in raising your body's oxygen level. The body is constantly producing a substance called "ATP" from our food. It has to keep producing it constantly, because we can't store much of it in the cells. The body is amazing, it can produce ATP in either an oxygen rich body environment, or in an environment without oxygen.

Usually we go along, "burning energy" from the ATP that is produced in the presence of oxygen. No problem... Suddenly we have to run very fast to grab a child out of the way of a speeding car! In that moment, or under similar important, or, athletic competitive situations, we can't breathe fast enough, to immediately process enough oxygen, to make this ATP out of an oxygen environment. So, the body, being equipped for survival, makes it anyway. The problem is, that this anaerobic formulation of ATP is *different* than the aerobic formulation. It has a much lower energy potential, and it leaves lactic acid behind in the muscles. Why is this a problem? Aside from reduced efficiency, lactic acid causes your muscles to quickly fatigue, and your strength and endurance to deplete rapidly. If you have a high tissue oxygen content, you produce more energy, last longer, and fatigue less. The amount of oxygen you can consume is called your "aerobic capacity". By exercising regularly, you can increase this capacity up to 30%.

THE SCIENCE OF BREATH

One of the first breath exercises I learned, was from a little book that was first published, in English, in 1904, by the Yogi Publication Society, and written by Yogi Ramacharaka. I have found it very educational. At one time, I practiced it regularly, and was able to develop an ability to swim underwater for a great distance. So, from personal experience, I can attest to it's ability to oxygenate the body. Athletes practicing this technique could increase their breathing capacity.

India's ancient culture has long been a storehouse of knowledge, often predating modern discoveries of the subtle workings of the body and atomic structure. To help their sincere spiritual seekers with their studies, the ancient spiritual teachers developed many very efficient ways to purify the body, which they considered the Temple of The Spirit.

BREATHING AND THE LIFE FORCE

The best all-around breathing exercises that I know of are found in the system known as The Ancient Science of Breath. This teaching gives us the "Complete Breath". While reading this, please do not equate this with hyperventilation, which is an excited state of taking in more oxygen than we need, on a short term basis, and with resistance.

My own very condensed version of these ancient Yogic practices and beliefs follows (paraphrased): Physical life is a series of breaths. Natural man breathes correctly, civilized man has contracted improper methods and attitudes of sitting, standing, and walking, which have robbed him of his birthright of natural and correct breathing. This has been a contributing factor in disease. Air contains more than oxygen, hydrogen, and nitrogen; it also carries what we can refer to as the Life Force. The Life Force, is closely linked to oxygen, and has electric, magnetic, and gravitic properties. Correct application of this treats disease, fear, worry, and the baser emotions.

The oxygen of the air comes in contact with the impure blood in the lungs. "Here a form of combustion takes place, and the blood takes up oxygen, and releases carbonic acid gas, generated from the waste products and poisonous matter, which have been gathered up by the blood, from all parts of the system. The blood, thus purified and oxygenated, is carried back to the heart, again rich, red, and bright, and laden with life-giving qualities and properties."

AVOID MOUTH BREATHING

Nostril breathing is far superior to mouth breathing, which should be avoided. The nostrils are an important filtering and straining system, purifying the air reaching the delicate organs. Breathing can be classified four ways:

1. High in the lungs (collarbone), requiring the most expenditure of energy and the least benefit; it is practiced, unconsciously, by most of us. You're probably doing it now.
2. Mid-lung (ribs).
3. Low in the lungs (diaphragmic, or deep).
4. The Complete Breath, which is far better.

DOING THE COMPLETE BREATH

The Complete breath contains all the best of the other three, with their shortcomings eliminated. The most important thing, is that it must be performed with *total relaxation*. Never strain against any set of muscles. You could learn this lying down, and once learned, do it sitting, standing, and then, all the time. Usually when we take a deep breath, we fill the upper part of our lungs, then the middle, then try and force some more air in deeper. Stop reading and try it now.....

The Complete Breath is performed in the opposite order, from the bottom up, and without force. Breathing only through the nose, imagine just below your intestines is the top section of an inflated balloon, which fills your body completely, in a large circle. Your stomach, lungs, and all internal organs rest on it. Attached to the center of this balloon top, is the end of a stick that extends through the center of your body, down between your legs and feet.

A friend of yours slowly pulls this stick down, as far as is comfortable, 90 degrees away from the soles of your feet, while you gently (but completely) push down from above, and all your internal organs and your lungs follow. Try it. Immediately, your lungs have to take in more air, to fill the vacuum. Mentally pull the stick way down, and still, totally relaxed, start to fill what feels like the very bottom of your stomach with air. When it's full, only then do you allow any air to start filling your upper stomach and lower ribs.

Now expand your chest the same way. In each case, you must physically expand (inflate) these areas. They should stretch out your body. Use your hands to feel the expansion at first: the diaphragm slowly pulls down, next, the stomach pushes out, next, the ribs expand. Then, the upper chest expands and rises, and when you think you're at the absolute limit, and can't fit in any more air, then you must momentarily hold this position, and shift your awareness to your ribs. Notice any areas that are resisting, and totally relax them, drawing in more air, and probably expanding another inch or two. I have always found there to be that last little bit, that I physically cannot expand, unless I melt the resistance mentally (through more relaxation). But once I do, it feels great.

COUNT

You are sequentially expanding a 360 degree balloon that starts at the bottom of your stomach, and ends at your neck. After you get the technique down, you could experiment with using you imagination to expand further. While inhaling, count slowly (mentally only), to see how long this expansion takes. Take as long as you possibly can. Once this is accomplished, you must (still remaining totally relaxed) hold all the air in your body for as long as you can, and start a new count. Then, slowly let the air out, counting again. Exhale everything in the reverse sequence: first top, then middle, then lower. All the while have your imagined friend push up, (in the reverse direction) on the imaginary stick. You will find yourself exhaling stale air that you didn't even know you had. Now, hold yourself with your lungs totally empty, as long as you can. Count this exhale/hold. Repeat the process. Do this for 20 minutes.

There are four movements. Inhale. Hold. Exhale. Hold. At first, you practice these four steps as distinct movements. This is not the idea, however, as this should be as a fluid, wavelike motion, which comes with practice. Try to extend your counts with each session. As an approximation, the inhale and exhale should be about equal, and the inhale hold, and exhale hold, less than that, & equal. 10-5-10-5, increasing with practice to 20-10-20-10 and beyond. If you have any trouble sustaining any of the four counts, lower the others to match it, while you slowly bring it up to their level. Balance is the object. Perhaps you could get to the point where all four counts are equal.

YOGIC USE OF TECHNIQUE

The Yogis would expand upon this exercise, to induce a state where they imagined themselves as separate from their bodies, and actually part of giving and receiving love, to and from everything. But for our purposes, it is enough to use this to increase our cellular oxygenation. The average person has a lung capacity of 250cc's, but with a few weeks of daily practice, it is possible to double it. The Yogis stated that - when the capacity reaches 750cc's - the intuitional powers develop more fully.

SPIRITUALITY AND PSYCHIC PHENOMENA LINKED TO OXYGENATION

Contemplative exercises, calm, heartfelt, non-intrusive prayer, relaxation techniques, and meditation, have been shown to reduce the body's need for oxygen. This, in effect, could be seen as increasing the cell environment oxygenation, as less energies are used to sustain stress, and more are then available, for normal cellular oxidation functions.

LAYING ON OF HANDS

I have also spoken with a physicist, who did a study of the "laying on of hands", and other psychic types of healing. He said they've found out by experiments, that some of the first effects of such methods were <u>increased oxygen</u> at the injury site, more than just from the warmth of the hands. This is logical, in that Nature always uses a great wisdom, and economy of effort. It always does the correct thing, in just the right amount, to restore balance when viewed in the big picture. So, the simplest thing would be to boost the oxygen levels. That way the already in place immune system gets enough building blocks to do the repair.

KARMA

Since I brought this area up, and because I don't want to be accused of advocating such practices, I'll share something that may help someone, although it's an aside to our topic of oxygenation. Physical health care professionals, working with physical methods, are serving a normal function in society. For the purposes of this discussion, they are not included in this following point: the reason I do not advocate the above practice, is, that it is

possible for a psychic "healer" to rob Soul (you) of an experience
needed in the classroom of suffering. The psychic "healer" may be
able to effect changes, but in the process, might incur the karma
of the disease, by this act of denying Soul an experience it needs.
Outcomes are always uncertain, when working with other than the
highest energies.

This is why I believe the best method, is not to try and
change anything by directing non-physical energies at a person, but
to raise your own consciousness as high as possible, and then
declare yourself merely available to do the Will of the Creator
(Your concept of The Divinity), for the good of the whole. If you
are used by it, for the Life Force to flow through, fine. If not,
fine. The technique is, to let The Creator decide, if and how, to
use the Life Force, not you. You see, this way, the error-laden
human mind stays out of the equation, and The Creator's Will is
done.

MUSICAL, SONIC, AND ARTISTIC THEORIES

We will now enter non-mainstream areas, that I will relate to
our oxygenation topic later on. If you think about it, in Rife's
work, we just saw that there is a whole world of life we've been
ignoring, only because our eyes don't see, that high up, the
frequency scale. What if we're also ignoring another whole world
of life that exists, just because our *ears* don't listen closely
enough? We see pictures of microscopes, but no super powered
microphones or *radio antennas* focused right down into the cells.
Do we know *everything* yet?

MUSIC FROM THE CELLS

A scientist in the late 1800's, John Keely, maintained that
every element has a main tone, or keynote. Groups of atoms and
compounds, combine to form this overall keynote and it's harmonics.
Because life is a process of creation, every living thing is
emitting frequencies. If you are not moving, just sitting there,
your brain is emitting the electrical impulses of living. The
electrons of the atoms in your body are orbiting around, and their
movement creates many vibrations, which results in creating sound.
The atoms of a cell are spinning in their own way, with each cell's
combined movement vibrating, or "singing", it's own note. All the
notes combine, to create the harmonious chorus of life. When a
cell is invaded by another organism, it's vibrational frequency and
electrical potentials change. It's like a chord struck on a piano.
Rather than the original chord, we now have added strange notes to
it. The unnatural invaders, or toxins, produce different additive
and subtractive frequencies and harmonics. They "sound different".

No longer vibrating the same tune as it's neighbors, the out
of sync, or infected area, or cell, stands out from the harmony of
it's neighbors, like a bad note on a piano. I suspect this might
have something to do with how our previously discussed ozone or
peroxide-created, free radical scavengers, only affect diseased
cells.

206

CELLULAR RADIO

A researcher measured the transmissions of the cellular DNA. He said they emit frequencies in the 1.9 to 2 megacycle range, in order to detect, by returning frequency-shifted echo, what type of protein is missing in the cell. This researcher is Gianni A. Dotto, who holds separate Ph.D.'s in: Nuclear physics, Electrical Engineering, & Mechanical Engineering. He has been granted two patents: #3,839,771, Oct. 8, 1974, the DOTTO RING, which is said to create the proper frequencies for the DNA, & patent #3,785,383, Jan 15, 1974, ELECTROSTATIC WAND. His lab is in Dayton, OH.

Dr. Dotto explained: our cells emit these waves by virtue of the fact that the DNA coil structure is a miniature antenna. The cell "listens" to how these frequencies (that it emits) are bouncing off everything around it, and notes any modification to the original waves. In the same way, this is how radar works. The returning waves are altered by striking something, the cell interprets this information, and targets an area for repair, or other adjustment, as long as the cell has enough life force itself. If the cell "hears" a returning signal, that is altered by injury or toxins, it gets a false "radar reading" of it's condition, and starts making adjustments, sometimes incorrect ones, and we say that it mutated. Now we are said to have a diseased cell.

There is a whole body of knowledge surrounding the theory that we can actually introduce perfect, low power (those little cells are delicate), radio emissions, into the cells. From transmitters outside the body. Please note, I said *low* power, very low power. It is thought to be theoretically possible, and is also ancedotaly reported, that: diseased cells can lock onto, or come into resonance with, corrected signals from an outside source. The cells then "think" the transmitted waves are their own returning waves, and they will repair themselves. This occurs, because the unnatural transmissions from disease are overridden. At the same time, the diseased cell's diminished life-force is "boosted" back to health, or normalcy, by the input waves. This is the basis of a device known as the Multi Wave Oscillator, which has been in use, in some hospitals in: France, Germany and Italy. Georges Lakhovsky held U.S. patent #1,962,565, on the MWO, and it is now in public domain. He said disease is a struggle between cell waves. If you pursue this area, be aware that there is some controversy around, that questions if the units built from current plans are as good as the original manufactured units. And, are the coincentric-ring, printed-circuit, flat-foil antennas as good as circular-metal, tubular antennas? Some say they all have beneficial effect.

Contact: B.S.R.F. P.O. Box 429-OT, Garberville, California 95440. They have 3 reports on the MWO. Super Science, PO Box 392-OT, Dayton, OH, 45409, they also sell reports. Mike Brown manufactures a MWO, based on the original design transmitter, given to Lakhovsky by Tesla. He also has a water oxygenator system using commercial oxygen. Mike Brown, Box 122-OT, San Marcos, CA, 92069. H&H Products P.O. Box 38092-OT, Shreveport, LA, 71133, also sells the MWO. $875.

SOUND AND LIGHT

Looking at this, from a non-technical viewpoint, the singing of certain Hymns, or the daily chanting practices of some monastic Christian orders, have been ancedotaly known to prevent disease. There's a story around, that when the monks of a certain monastery maintained their hard ascetic life-styles, but stopped chanting for hours every day, many of them soon got sick. They were puzzled by this at first, but someone made the connection, and they reinstituted the daily chants. Once they resumed chanting, no one was getting ill. The only thing changed was the elimination and then eventual restoration of the daily chanting disciplines. The deep breathing encountered by singing and chanting, forces more oxygen into the lungs, and the vibrations that the sounds set up, are like the aforementioned radio waves. Other religions actively teach that by chanting certain sounds, phrases, or "mantras", that they can effect changes at the cellular level. For more proof, go to Tibet, and visit some Tibetan monasteries that have been hidden away for ages. That's probably a little too ambitious for you, right now, especially since the Red Chinese control much of the Tibetan countryside. However, I'm sure that there are Buddhist and Tibetan monks teaching somewhere near you. Both chant daily, and you can see this in action.

This chanting, is an example of using our creative powers to produce sound (a group of frequencies and harmonics), and resonating them into the cells during singing, or vibrating the body. Some say that: the chord C-E-G#, followed by C#-F-A, then D-F#-A#, then D#-G-B, and repeated, continuously, would be using trines of harmony. How about, at the same time, taking harmonious colored lights (more frequencies and harmonics) and shining them onto (introducing their waves into) the body and it's cells? There are many newspaper accounts of UFO abductees ancedotaly reporting that they were healed, by having colored lights shone on them. Trined colors: red-green-violet, orange-turquoise-purple, yellow-blue-magenta, and lemon-indigo-scarlet. This is part of music and color therapy, or what's called, sound and light healing.

REMOVING INTERFERENCE

Let's put this all together, and return to our theme. If you clean up the toxins, "crud", and other unoxidized or "unburnt" products of your metabolism, so that these wastes can no longer surround the cells, interfering with, and mutating the cell wave emissions, then once again, the natural harmonious music is sent and received by the DNA. With the correct information, the codes that have been stored in our DNA since birth, being sent and received, the cells can repair themselves. Do you remember what the methods is, that many of the experts in this book proclaim to be effective, in cleaning up the body's unnatural, vibration altering toxins? Yep, OXYGENATION!

This information is given to you, to show that there might be a lot of work to be done, in exploring Sympathetic Vibratory Physics and many other avenues of life. A great source of related topics is the newsletter: "Sympathetic Vibratory Physics" put out by Dale Pond at Delta Spectrum Research, Inc. 4810-OT Airport Rd., Colorado Springs, Colorado 80916

FACTORS BEYOND PHYSICAL BALANCE

My editors all warned me to leave this section out, they said I sound like I'm selling my concept of The Creator. I'm not. I appreciate their concern, but I never was one to hold back what I consider a necessary ingredient. One of the problems with science, is that it often takes our precious humanity out of the equation.

I'm leaving this section in because I am positive that there is more to disease than the strictly physical mechanisms. I am not selling anything. I am sharing the fact that something I discovered is available to you too, just like when I told you about all the places you could go to obtain oxygenation resources. Any attempt by me to impose my personal beliefs upon you would be a violation of your space, and spiritual law.

There is no single "cure" that works on every patient every time. The reason, is simple: unless all the physical, emotional, mental, & spiritual causes of the illness are removed, or balanced out, the illness may hang on, or have a chance of returning.

In this book, "Oxygen Therapies" I have tried to show you the necessity of reversing the cellular hydrogenation process, and effecting detoxification by oxygenation, if optimum health is your goal. It has been said, that there are ultimately no factors limiting life, except from what we do to ourselves, or allow into our bodies and thoughts. Theoretically, if everyone lived in harmony with others, and the environment, and if we kept our cells "sparkling" clean and properly nourished in the exact proper proportions, both with food, and the Life Force, we could extend our physical lives indefinitely.

As you know, that's a little tough to do right now, due to our planet's present stage of evolutionary development. What we can try to do, is increase our survival factors by degree. Every step we take towards universal balance goes to our credit. If you can only do a little, then you're still better off than before, and probably a little healthier, and nicer to be around.

To treat man's "other than physical" ailments, various people and groups, possessing differing degrees of illumination, have devised or evolved ways to try and help us. This help ranges from getting a friend's advice, to attending the local church service, or belonging to an informal, or organized, educational/discovery group. The best place I have found to ultimately get the most reliable advice is deep within myself, in that "calm, expansive place". All the world's great teachers have told us to "go to the Temple Within", for indeed, that is where our small selves meet The Creator.

This making of the conscious connection, from our outer lives to our inner worlds, can be enhanced by study, practice, and affiliation with those who have realized this process, and now consciously operate within it. The side benefits we get are increased emotional and metabolic balance, and physical harmony. The diversity of the paths and teachings becoming available to us is increasing, as our planet's consciousness elevates. This consciousness elevation is due to a number of factors. A major factor is the technology & communications revolution, or, "explosion". Another possible factor is that our solar system is transiting a new area of cosmic energies, or, maybe it's just "time" for it to happen.

All paths have something to offer, and each is a step toward what I believe to be our Ultimate Goal: returning to The Creator as conscious co-workers with It. Some readers might be curious about my personal preference. This author, after studying many of the world's phenomena, has come to the personal conclusion that his favorite body of knowledge is a teaching called Eckankar. "Eck" is the Life Force, and "ankar" means "study of". Many methods work, and no one has all the answers. However, after much searching, I settled on this teaching. In my opinion, the Eck teachers offer me the most efficient methods of restoring emotional, mental, and spiritual balance. A necessary part of any permanent change in the direction of health.

The area of spiritual preference is sometimes touchy to speak of, since it is usually emotionally charged. I sincerely hope no offense is taken by anyone, simply because I answered a question by stating my personal preference. So that my position is clearly understood, I will restate my main point: there are many different paths and many different people. Any may be right for you, personally, at any point in time. The ECK teachings have worked well for me. I am not an official spokesperson of Eckankar, and the opinions expressed anywhere in this book are mine, and not necessarily those of Eckankar. For further information on Eckankar, their office can be reached at: (612)544-0066, or write: P.O.Box 27300-OT, Minneapolis, MN, 55427.

That's what's great about this country, we always have the freedom to choose our own methods of individually approaching The Divinity. For example: I have some very healthy and happy friends who practice Kriya Yoga. One of them healed his freshly broken rib, overnight, by entering into what he called a "Super Conscious" state, wherein existed, no such imperfections like broken bones. He came out of it healed. He went to the Temple Within. The break, and repair within 24 hours, were verified by X-rays. I have met Sufis that had such good auras, that they were a joy to stand next to. I have studied the lives of Christian, Jewish, Sufi, and Buddhist Saints. Followers of their ways are blessed, and have wonderful lives. There are others, as well. The point is, not what label we put on It, but always: how well are you practicing "The Presence of The Divinity" right now? Or, if you have a personal cosmology that disagrees with the whole idea of there being any form of Creator, ask yourself how well you are living by your own personal code of ethics. How we answer these questions, may go a long way toward determining our health.

REQUEST, CONCLUSION, AND SUMMARY

Please do us all a favor, OK? If you ever try any of the products or methods in this book, or ones like them, please write me, and tell me what happened. Whether or not I will have the time and circumstance to answer is unknown, but that won't be important. Getting the input is what's important. I am establishing a record of any oxygenation experiences, for the benefit of The Whole. Please do not ask me any medical questions, as I am not a doctor.

Why is it some people don't respond to _any_ treatments, no matter what they are? Some wait too long before investigating alternatives. Their disease has destroyed so much tissue that the bodily defenses can't do the repair. Unfortunately, some of the alternative clinics have had to refuse treatment to cancer patients who have had extensive radiation or chemotherapy damage. This stops a clinic from being blamed for damage done elsewhere. Some don't respond because they believe they really **need** to suffer, it's a psychological thing. The patient might subconsciously want punishment to satisfy guilt over a questionable previous action. Maybe the sufferer has even been conditioned to "know" they are really "no good", or a similar control factor is in place. There is also the condition of being hurt somehow, but never really letting go of the experience. Keeping dead images alive, the energy goes back in instead of coming out. These are a few of the common reasons to continually self-create illness.

I mentioned control factors. Some of us have been so conditioned into letting experts tell us what to do, that we've forgotten who's in charge. How many opinions are formed, and how many lives are lived, based upon the certainty that the only truth around is disseminated by television?

We're the only real experts on our own lives. Only listening to influences outside of ourselves is error. Error leads to imbalance. Imbalance may turn to disease. having said that, don't go too far on your own. Remember, experts and friends are a wonderful resource, and should be learned from, and trusted, when appropriate. The point is to strike a balance between the inner and outer influences. A slave is totally outer directed. A madman totally mind directed. A balanced person regularly dips into their inner well of creativity, sees how all of life is connected in harmony, and acts with responsibility as a caretaker of that knowledge.

If, after reading this book, you are still unsure about the health benefits that will evolve from oxygenating a deficient body properly, then all I can do is strongly encourage you to track down the experts, companies, and historical sources listed in this book yourself. That's where it all starts, with you taking action.

Thank you for reading my book. I hope you were informed, and entertained. After all my research, there is but one thing I can conclude:

WE ALL HAVE A LOT LEFT TO DISCOVER.

ED McCABE'S "OXYGEN THERAPIES"
INDEPENDENT JOURNALISM
ORDER FORM

NAME_____

ADDRESS1_____

ADDRESS2_____

CITY_____STATE_____ZIP_____

ORDER DATE_____ SHIP VIA_____

CREDIT CARD TYPE_____ CARD NUMBER_____ EXPIRATION_____

AUTHORIZATION SIGNATURE _____

QTY.   *INTRODUCTORY PUBLICATIONS - ALL DISEASES*   TOTAL

BOOK: "OXYGEN THERAPIES A NEW WAY OF APPROACHING DISEASE" - BESTSELLER!
THE CLASSIC TEXT WITH PAGES OF MEDICAL REFERENCES $18 ea. $

AUDIO TAPE: "AN INTRODUCTION TO OXYGEN THERAPIES"
EXPO RECORDING WITH SPECIAL PRIVATE COMMENTS ADDED $15 ea. $

VIDEO TAPE: "OXYGEN THERAPIES INTRODUCTORY VIDEO - FIRST AUSTRALIAN TRIP"
ED'S SLIDE SHOW OF ALL THE THERAPIES - 2 HOURS. $25 ea. $

SPECIALTY PUBLICATIONS

NEW REPORT!: "O_3 vs. AIDS" (OZONE CHRONOLOGY -INCL. CANCER). 40 pgs. ABBREVIATED
HISTORY OF US MEDICAL OZONE RESEARCH AND SUPPRESSION $17.50 ea. $

AUDIO TAPE: "BREAKING THE OZONE SILENCE" SIDE 1 - AUDIO VERSION OF
1992 CHRONOLOGY, SIDE 2 - HISTORIC KPFK INTERVIEW $15 ea. $

NEW VIDEO!: "OZONE THERAPIES, CANCER AND AIDS" - 2ND AUSTRALIAN LECTURE SERIES
BRISBANE 2 HOURS 40 MINUTES, INCLUDES ACTUAL TESTIMONIALS $29 ea. $

(Aove pricing incldes shipping, FL residents add tax)   GRAND TOTAL $

THE FAMILY NEWS INC.
9845 N.E. 2ND AVE. MIAMI SHORES, FL 33138
800/284-6263   305/759-8710   FAX 305/759-8689